The Back Pain Solution

Unlocking the Spinal Code

Dr. Douglas Jay Taber

Disclaimer

The information in this book is intended for educational use only and should not be construed as medical advice. Do not try self-diagnosis or attempt self-treatment without consulting a medical professional or qualified practitioner. Do not undertake any self-treatment while you are undergoing a prescribed course of medical treatment without first seeking professional advice. Always seek professional help if your symptoms persist or worsen over time. Although every attempt is made to ensure that the information presented here is accurate, neither the publisher nor author will be liable for errors or omissions in the information presented, or any injuries that result therefrom.

Center Path Publishing
14859 Embry Path
Apple Valley, MN 55124

The paper used in this publication meets the minimum requirements of the American National Standards for Information Services - Permanence of Paper for Printed Library Materials, ANSI Z39.48-1984.

Library of Congress Cataloging-in-Publication Data

Taber, Douglas Jay.
The back pain solution : unlocking the spinal code / by Douglas Jay Taber.
p. cm.
Includes index.
ISBN-13: 978-1-933889-04-7 (alk. paper)
1. Spinal cord—Wounds and injuries—Popular works. 2. Spinal cord—Wounds and injuries—Treatment—Popular works. I. Title.
RA645.S66T33 2006
617.4'82044—dc22

2006010506

I would like to dedicate this book to my beautiful wife, Jennifer.
To the world, you might be one person.
But to me, you are the world.

Acknowledgements

"The master in the art of living makes little distinction between his work and play, his labor and his leisure, his mind and his body, his information and his recreation, his love and his religion.

He hardly knows which is which. He simply pursues his vision of excellence at whatever he does, leaving others to decide whether he is working or playing. To him, he is always doing both."

- James Michener, American author

I would first and foremost like to thank God for the blessings that He has bestowed upon my life. Without Him, nothing would be possible.

I also want to thank you for purchasing and reading this book. The many hours I have spent producing this work were fueled by the thought that others would learn from the information in these pages.

I want to thank my mother, Julie, who has taught me the importance of unconditional love and compassion for others, and my father, Douglas, who, through his words and actions, has led by example in teaching me the value of hard work, passion for life, and the pursuit of individualism.

My gratitude is also extended to my teachers and professors who taught me that in science as in life, every answer leads to a new question.

I also want to thank all of the people who were instrumental in the preparation and publishing of this book, including Dr. Todd Berntson at Center Path Publishing. My sincere gratitude is also extended to Michael Vallone, the talented artist who designed my book cover, and to Terry Cribbs, master photographer, for his contributions to this book. My appreciation goes out to Agatina Vallone for her editorial input. Thank you to Brittany Spritzer for modeling for the exercise photos.

Thank you to my office staff, LeAnn, Prema, Brittany, and Jennifer. You have been a wonderfully loyal and supportive group. Your enthusiasm and dedication are treasured and appreciated.

And finally, my sincere appreciation is extended to my patients: current, past, and future. It has truly been, and will continue to be, my honor and privilege to play a small role in your lives and to share in the experience of helping you regain and maintain your greatest resource: your health.

Thanks, everyone!

Table of Contents

I

Introduction

"The doctor of the future will give no medicine, but will interest his patients in the care of the human frame, in diet, and in the cause and prevention of disease."

- Thomas Edison

I vividly remember my younger days growing up in Central New York. As a child, I was always interested in becoming a doctor. My great-grandfather Malcolm would call me "doc," convinced that someday I would become a doctor. My parents would regularly buy me the latest doctor's kit from the local store or catalog.

In my childhood years, I was often plagued with illness and frequent trips to the doctor for recurrent bronchitis, asthma, and stomachaches, which kept me under a physician's care for the better part of my pre-teenage years. Through the constant poking, prodding, injections, and medications, I slowly lost my desire to become a doctor. At this young age, I was already disillusioned and disappointed in this approach to restoring health.

As a teenager, I became active in various sports and weight lifting. My health and outlook on life slowly improved as I took an interest in diet and exercise. In school, I would always smile with pride when my dad, an avid exerciser, would go running by my classroom window in his shorts and sneakers during his lunch break. "That's my dad," I would think. "Where's everybody else's dad? Are they exercising right now? Probably not."

I wanted to be like that. I wanted to guard, protect, and prioritize my health above all other possessions. I would use the home gym equipment dad had purchased to try new exercises that I'd read about or learned from my uncles Peter and Tony, both weight lifters and police officers.

As a teenager, I would read anatomy books and muscle magazines to learn about muscular development and nutrition. I just could not get enough information on the latest in human performance. I would order protein powders and go to the vitamin store at the mall to test out the latest nutritional supplements I would read about. I was hooked on a lifestyle of health and fitness.

In 1993 at the age of 22, I injured my low back while shoveling snow. After several days of masking the pain with Tylenol, I was frustrated and concerned. I could not get out of bed, let alone exercise.

At the suggestion of a co-worker, I made an appointment with a chiropractor. Although I had never seen one before, I knew that one of my favorite bodybuilders, Dr. Franco Columbu, was a chiropractor, and had treated Arnold Schwarzenegger. So, how bad could it be?

The following day, I showed up at the doctor's office, filled out my paperwork, and was taken into an exam room. I remember asking myself, "Where are all the posters, pens, and brochures with the drug company and medication names on them? Why do all the pictures on the wall have healthy messages on them?" It was completely foreign, yet oddly comforting, to be in an office with such a healing atmosphere.

The doctor entered the room and asked me a series of questions about my problem. He then evaluated my movement, checked my reflexes, and explained to me that I had sprained my lumbar spine. He showed me a spine model and some charts to help explain what was happening.

The doctor helped me to a table where I lay for 15-minutes with a heat pack and a machine with four pads that "massaged" my back. He then put me through a series of slow and gentle stretches and laid me on my side. The area where I had hurt for over a week made a small "popping" sound, and like an immediate release of pressure, my pain was gone. The doctor then showed me three stretches I could do at home, and explained to me how I could avoid a relapse.

No pills. No needles. No surgery. No follow-up appointment was even suggested; the doctor told me to call him if I was not better in 3-4 days.

My pain was gone immediately and, to my excitement, did not return. Because the problem had been explained to me, I was armed with the knowledge of what was wrong and what could be done for it, and how I could avoid re-injury while maintaining an active lifestyle.

By the end of the week, I was back at the gym. For the next several months, I read everything I could about chiropractic care and natural remedies. Whenever I had a headache or aches and pains, the chiropractor became the first person I would consult.

After finishing my undergraduate training and receiving my Bachelor of Science degree, my interest in the workings of the human body, diet, and exercise, combined with my enjoyment of problem solving and a desire to help people, culminated in the pursuit of a career as a Doctor of Chiropractic.

I am a Doctor of Chiropractic because I honor the inborn potential of everyone to be truly healthy. I wish to assist with healing rather than intrude; to free rather than control. I choose to care for the patient with the disease, not the disease. Everyday, I am confronted with painful and challenging spinal syndromes. Everyday, I am able to see miracles and offer hope.

What is "Unlocking the Spinal Code"?

Unlocking the spinal code means learning about the wonders of the human body and the fact that the nervous system is the master controller of every system in the body. It is about understanding the medical fact that a body of growing evidence suggests that many conditions can be traced back to spinal dysfunction.

When confronted with back or neck pain, unlocking the spinal code involves understanding your treatment options and integrating the safest, most effective ways to manage and prevent pain. By using the right formula of conventional treatment methods (medication, injections, pain management techniques, etc.) as well as more conservative options (diet, exercise, chiropractic, etc.), you can unlock your own unique spinal code and regain and maintain a healthy spine and nervous system.

The literal meaning of the word "doctor" is "teacher." The goal of this book is to share with you life-changing lessons and help to clear any confusion in an ever-changing health care environment. My hope is that these lessons will serve to teach you to understand true health and to live free of pain.

Each of the book's twelve chapters covers important topics that are relevant to your health. In the first chapter, you will learn the basics of how your body works. This may be the most important chapter in the whole book because the better you understand how your body works, the better health choices you can make. The remaining chapters include information about back and neck pain, headaches and whiplash injuries, as well as a variety of diagnostic and therapeutic options that are available to help you manage or completely eliminate your pain.

1

The Human Body

"The human body represents the actions of three laws: spiritual, mechanical and chemical, united as one triune. As long as there is a perfect union of these three, there is health."

-D.D. Palmer, the founder of chiropractic

Starting at conception, the human body begins to take shape, beginning with the development of a long cylindrical tube that forms the spinal cord. From this cord, tiny bumps begin to form that make up the internal organs as well as the arms and legs. This process continues, seemingly by magic, for nine months until a fully formed human being emerges. As long as all of the organs function in a tightly controlled balance, the child will continue to thrive and grow into a healthy adult.

While you sit calmly reading this, your body is bristling with activity. The trillions of cells that make up your body are busy at work performing thousands of delicately balanced processes that make your life possible. The brilliance with which your body controls this profoundly complex dance of chemistry is truly awe-inspiring. As long as your body is able to keep the dance going, you remain healthy and vibrant. However, if there is a disruption in any of the body's processes, the entire system loses its ability to perform correctly and disease emerges.

Such is the miracle of life. Our anatomy is the structure that makes up our body's assets, while our physiology is the infinite amount of interrelated functions our body processes to keep us adapting to our ever-changing environment. Having a good understanding of and an appreciation for your anatomy and physiology can help you create a new level of confidence and trust in yourself and your body. The best way for you to build your health is to understand the assets of your body and know how to best protect them each and every day.

The body's ability to regulate and control the delicate balance of all of the necessary life processes is called "homeostasis." The term *homeostasis* is derived from the Greek words for "same" and "steady." It refers to the way the body acts to maintain a stable internal balance. For example, your body works to maintain a carefully regulated internal temperature of 98.6 degrees. If you go outside on a warm day and begin to work, your body will begin to sweat in an effort to keep your temperature stable. You may also begin to breathe deeper in an effort to keep your tissues supplied with oxygen during a period of increased demand, such as during intense exercise.

Disease and disability result whenever the body is stressed beyond its ability to maintain homeostasis. This stress can come from several sources including interference or irritation of the nervous system, trauma, poor diet, lack of exercise, or excessive emotional stress. In this chapter, you will learn about the systems in your body that are necessary for maintaining health.

Digestive System

When we eat such things as bread, meat, and vegetables, they are not in a form that the body can use. Everything that we eat and drink must be broken down into smaller molecules before they can be absorbed and used by the body. This process is called digestion.

The digestive system includes the digestive tract and its accessory organs, which process food into molecules that can be absorbed and utilized by the cells of the body. Food is broken down, bit by bit, until the molecules are small enough to be absorbed and the waste products are eliminated. The digestive tract, also called the alimentary canal or gastrointestinal (GI) tract, includes the mouth, esophagus, stomach, small intestine, and large intestine.

As long as this system works correctly, the nutrients you consume are able to be extracted and absorbed into the bloodstream to be delivered to your individual cells. The digestive system is the means by which you get all of the individual nutrients that are needed for health. Every single molecule in your entire body arrived there in the same way - at some point in the recent past you ate it. This is an important concept to remember because if your diet does not include everything that your body needs, you will lose some of the richness of your health. Consuming food is much like depositing money into your checking account. If you don't have enough resources there, you can't afford to keep fixing your house.

Cardiovascular System

The cardiovascular system is sometimes called the circulatory system. It consists of the heart, which is a muscular pumping device, and a closed system of vessels called arteries, veins, and capillaries. The role of the cardiovascular system in maintaining homeostasis is the transportation of nutrients and oxygen from the digestive system to all of the cells in the body, as well as the transportation of waste and carbon dioxide to be eliminated.

As long as your cardiovascular system works correctly, your body has an enormous capacity to adapt to just about any external demand. For example, when you begin to exercise, your heart pumps faster and your blood pressure increases in order to supply more oxygen and nutrients to your tissues. When you are cold, your blood vessels constrict in some areas of the body – the back of your arm, for instance – in an effort to conserve heat. When your body is injured, the blood vessels open up to allow white blood cells to enter the area to fight infection and speed healing.

Unfortunately, the cardiovascular system is the one that fails most often due to an unhealthy lifestyle. Heart disease is the number one cause of death in the United States and is also responsible for tragic disability in millions of Americans. The vast majority of heart disease is completely avoidable by making some simple lifestyle changes – exercise being the most important. The key phrase when it comes to your cardiovascular health is "use it or lose it." If you don't exercise and work out your cardiovascular system, you will lose it.

Immune System

Every minute of the day, we are exposed to dangerous bacteria, viruses, fungi, and the development of cancerous cells that, if allowed to grow, would result in illness or death. In fact, the bacteria and viruses living in and on our body outnumber our own cells. What keeps these invaders in check is the immune system.

When your immune system is compromised due to improper diet, stress, trauma, lack of exercise, spinal disorders, or for any other reason, you lose some of your ability to eliminate the harmful cells and invaders in your body, resulting in disease. Just like with your body's other systems, your lifestyle choices have a profound impact on how well your immune system functions.

The Neuromusculoskeletal System

The neuromusculoskeletal system is really three distinct systems that work as one coordinated unit: 1) the bones and joints (skeletal system), 2) the muscles, and 3) the nervous system. The neuromusculoskeletal system is by far the largest system in the body, comprising between 60% - 75% of your total body mass. It is also the most prone to injuries, dysfunction, and pain. Understanding how each of these systems work will provide you with the information to make better treatment and lifestyle choices and to live your life free from pain and disability.

The Bones and Joints

The human skeleton is made up of more than 200 bones that are connected by joints. Your bones are responsible for creating your body's general shape, and they serve to protect your internal organs and to manufacture blood cells. Each of your bones is made up of two compounds: a protein meshwork of collagen and a salt of calcium called hydroxyapatite.

The collagen fibers which make up the basic structure of your bones give them a great deal of resilience and resistance to breaking when twisted, bent, or impacted. It is actually the loss of this collagen meshwork and not just a loss of calcium that is responsible for the bone weakness associated with conditions such as osteoporosis. The other component of bone, hydroxyapatite, is a crystalline calcium salt which is integrated into the collagen meshwork. Hydroxyapatite is responsible for giving the bones rigidity and resistance to crushing under pressure.

Bones can be compared to steel-reinforced concrete, where the collagen acts much like the steel meshwork in the concrete, and the hydroxyapatite acts much like the concrete which surrounds the steel. Together they form a very tough, resilient, and rigid framework upon which the rest of the body is supported. Because your bones are rigid and do not bend, you would not be able to move if it were not for your joints.

Joints are much more than simply a place where the ends of two bones meet. They are very complicated systems of ligaments, tendons, membranes, fluid, and cartilage that allow the bones to move in a smooth, stable, and controlled way. Joints are designed in a wide variety of ways depending on their function and the particular stresses they have to endure. For example, the joints between your sternum (breastbone) and your ribs are simple joints consisting only of fibrous collagen. They are designed to be simple because the front part of your rib cage does not have to move very much in relation to your sternum. The shoulder joint, on the other hand, is an extremely complex joint that requires a whole host of muscles, ligaments, and tendons all working in concert with each other in order to move properly. If any one of the muscles or other structures of the shoulder are damaged, pain, instability, or loss of function may result.

Muscles

There are more than 650 muscles in your body which have only one purpose – to create movement. While your bones are what give your body its framework, the muscles are what give your body motion. There are more than three times the number of muscles in your body as there are bones, and each one of these muscles fills a particular role in creating movement. Like bones, your muscles also contain a lot of collagen for strength and resilience. Instead of calcium salts, muscles contain a specialized type of cell which has the unique ability to contract when stimulated by the nervous system.

There are actually three types of muscle in the body - smooth muscle, cardiac muscle, and striated muscle (also called skeletal muscle). Smooth muscle is found surrounding the organs of the digestive tract as well as the arteries. In the digestive tract, smooth muscle is responsible for moving the food we eat through our digestive system, while the smooth muscle which surrounds the arteries helps the regulation of blood flow throughout the body. Unlike skeletal muscles, smooth muscles are involuntary muscles, meaning that we do not have conscious control over them.

Cardiac muscle, as its name implies, is found only in the heart. What differentiates cardiac muscle from all other muscle in the body is the fact that it rhythmically contracts on its own, regardless of stimulation by the nervous system. As a matter of fact, if two independent cardiac cells, each rhythmically contracting to their own beat, are put in contact with each other, they will begin beating in unison.

The third type of muscle is skeletal muscle. This is the type of muscle that we can consciously control and the type of muscle that is of most interest to us because it is the type of muscle responsible for our posture and movement. Every skeletal muscle attaches to at least two different bones. As they contract, they draw the bones together using the joints as hinges.

Take for example the elbow joint. Compared to some of the other joints in the body such as the shoulder or hip, the elbow is a relatively simple hinge joint. Yet there are more than a dozen muscles which cross the elbow joint, all of which contribute to the elbow's normal movement. If any of these muscles do not fire in a highly coordinated fashion, or if some of the muscles are tighter or weaker than they should be, abnormal joint function and pain will likely result.

Abnormal posture and joint motion resulting from weak, spastic, or uncoordinated muscles is very common, especially in people who work at a desk all day. Since muscles become weaker unless they are exercised, it is important for good muscular health to include some form of resistance exercise as part of your daily routine.

The Nervous System "The Master Control Center"

The nervous system is made up of trillions of highly-specialized individual nerve cells, each of which communicate with hundreds or thousands of other nerve cells through tiny electrical pulses, and is comprised of two major systems. The first is the central nervous system, which includes your brain and spinal cord, and the other is called the peripheral nervous system, which includes the nerves that run from your spine to all areas of the body.

The nervous system is called the master control center, as it is responsible for the control of all major body functions including our senses, movement and balance, as well as the regulations of all body functions.

There are three types of nerves. These are called pain, or sensory nerves, motor nerves, and postural nerves, or more correctly, proprioceptors. Pain nerves do just what their name implies - they allow us to feel pain. Whenever something in our body hurts, it is because the pain nerves in the area are being stimulated and are sending signals to the brain to create the sensation of pain.

Motor nerves are responsible for controlling movement by stimulating muscles to contract. The fact that you are able to hold this book in your hands right now is because these motor nerves are contracting the muscles in your hands and arms. If these nerves aren't able to function correctly, it can result in weakness or paralysis in the muscles they control.

The third type of nerve is the proprioceptor, or what we will simply call the postural nerves. These nerves are responsible for sending information to the brain about where your body is and what it's doing. For example, if you close your eyes and hold your arm out to your side, you can tell exactly where your arm is even though you can't see it because the postural nerves of the arm and upper back tell the brain where your arm is. Many people have discovered what happens when their postural nerves aren't working correctly after they have had too much to drink. Alcohol partially disrupts the function of your cerebellum and postural nerves, making it difficult to touch your finger to your nose when your eyes are closed or walk a straight line with your eyes open.

The Spine

The human spine is a column of up to 34 bones called vertebrae, separated by tough fibrous pads called spinal discs (or intervertebral discs).

The spine is divided into five areas: the top seven vertebrae make up the cervical region (neck); below the neck are twelve thoracic vertebrae to which your twelve pairs of ribs attach; the low back region is made up of five lumbar vertebrae; below the lumbar region, there are five fused vertebrae that make up the sacrum; and finally, at the very base of the spine is the group of three fused vertebrae called the coccyx. On either side of the sacrum are the two bones of the pelvis.

The Spinal Vertebrae

Each vertebra consists of a vertebral body, which is a large oval-shaped solid block of bone, and a vertebral arch, which is located on the back of the vertebral body and creates the space through which the spinal cord runs. The vertebral body provides about 70% of all the structural support of the spine.

The Spinal Canal and Vertebral Arch

Directly in back of the vertebral body is an opening called the spinal canal. When all of the bones are stacked on top of each other, one continuous canal is formed. This is where the spinal cord runs from the brain down to all of the areas of the body.

Surrounding the spinal canal is the bony vertebral arch. Attached to the arch are a pair of joints called facet joints, and three bony protrusions called processes. The facet joints act as links holding the vertebrae together and strengthening the

The Regions of Your Spine

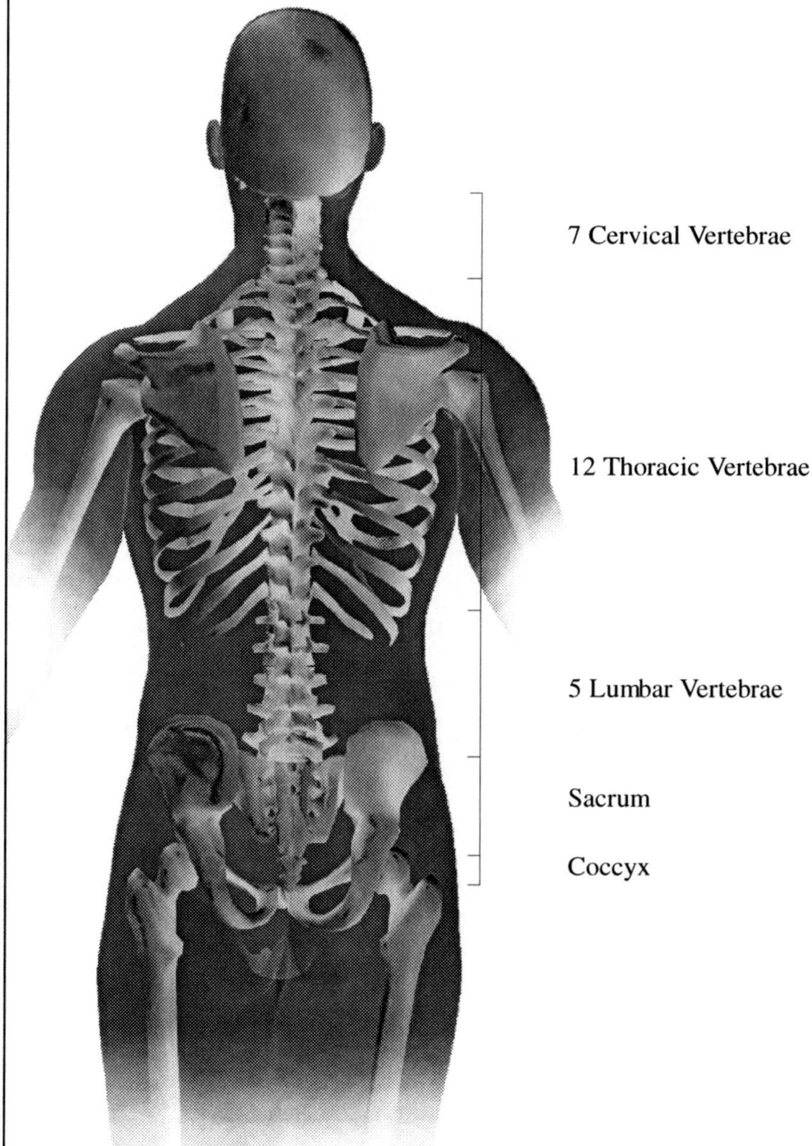

spine. They also bear 30% of the structural support of the spine.

The process located in the center of the arch is called the spinous process. These are the bony bumps that you can feel running down the center of your back. On either side of the spinous process are the two transverse processes. The processes act as anchor points for ligaments and muscles necessary for movement.

The Facet Joints

The facet joints play a large role in restricting the way in which two adjacent vertebrae move in relation to each other. For example, in the cervical spine (neck), the facet joints are oriented in such a way as to allow a considerable degree of rotation, whereas the facet joints in the lumbar spine (low back) are oriented in a way that restricts rotation. A simple experiment of turning your head from side to side and then trying to twist your low back to the same degree shows the effect that facet joints have on the movement of the spine.

The Intervertebral Discs

Each vertebra is attached to two adjacent spinal vertebrae with a disc between them. These discs, technically called intervertebral discs, are thick pads of fibrocartilage that act as shock

Basic Structures of the Spine

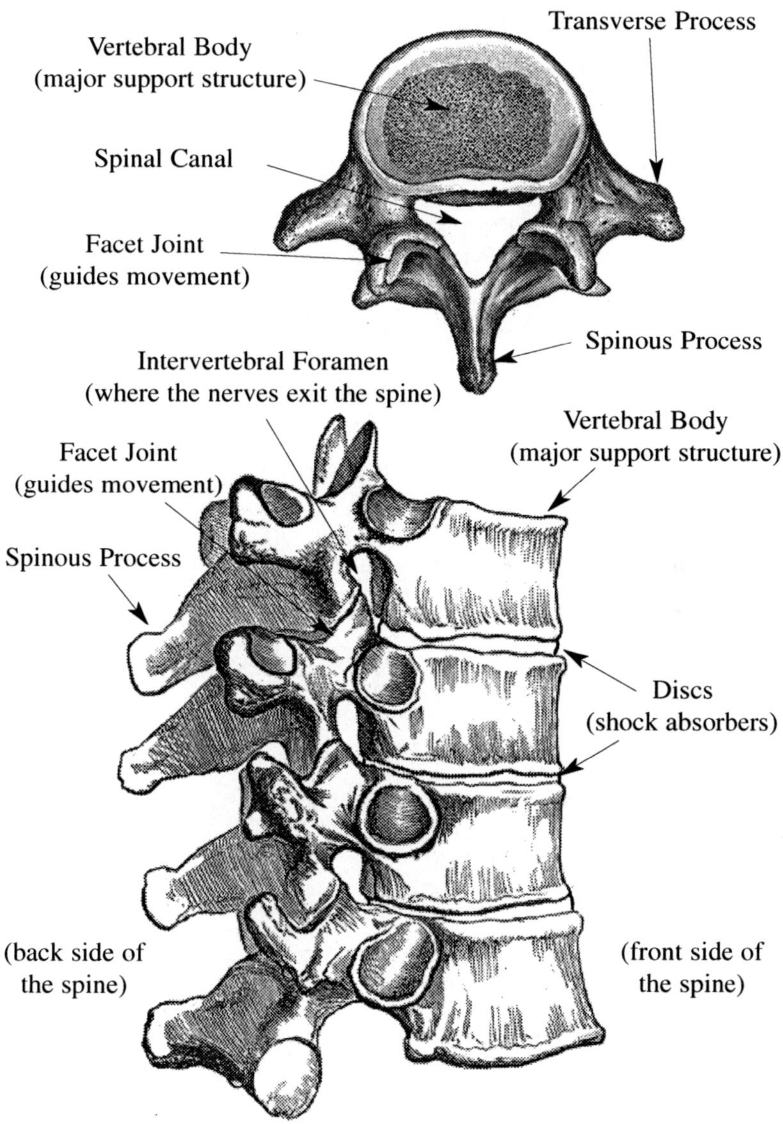

absorbers and give the spine its ability to flex and twist. The disc itself is kind of like a jelly-filled donut. It has an outer fibrous portion called the annulus, and a soft jelly-like center called the nucleus pulposis.

The Spinal Cord

The spine forms the protective housing for the spinal cord, which begins at the brain stem (back of the skull) and extends like a wire down the length of the spine. Ultimately, the spinal cord sends out nerve branches that send and receive signals to and from every cell in the body. The close relationship between the spine and the spinal cord means that damage to any of the discs or vertebrae can also affect the spine or portion of the spinal cord associated with it, causing pain or abnormal function of the structures innervated by the affected area.

Between each pair of vertebrae and behind the discs, there is a small space where the nerves exit from the spinal cord and run to all of the areas of the body. These spaces are called the vertebral foramen. *Foramen* is a medical term that simply means "hole."

The Ligaments

The joints in the spine are held together by tough, flexible bands of fiber called ligaments. In conjunction with the facet joints, the ligaments help to keep the spine in one piece. There

The Spine and Spinal Cord

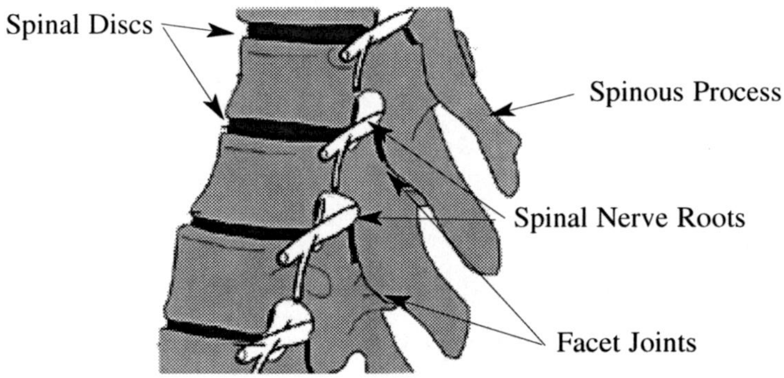

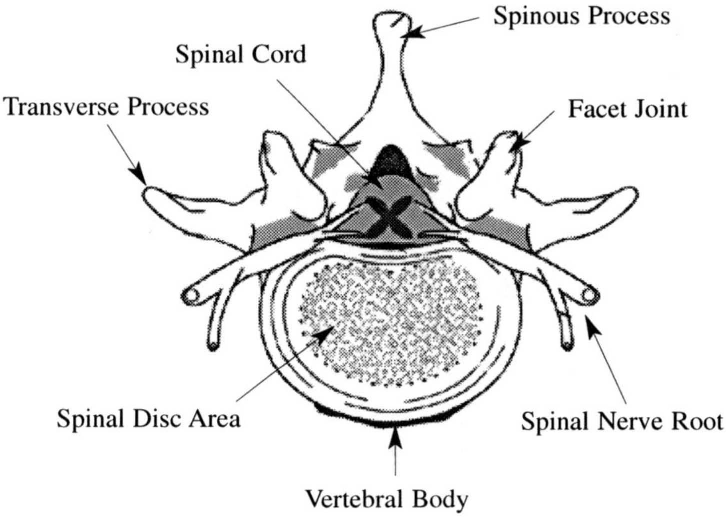

are four long ligaments that run down the entire length of the spine, as well as ligaments around each facet joint. Joint movement is important to keep the ligaments from becoming stiff. For this reason, regular physical activity is important to ensure that you maintain flexibility in the spine.

The Muscles

Muscles attach to the bony extensions of the vertebrae and provide movement in the spine by contracting in a highly coordinated way. Muscles tend to work in pairs, each pulling the bones across a joint in the opposite direction, and are important for stabilizing and strengthening the spine, as well as for providing movement. Like ligaments, muscles are also important for absorbing shock and releasing it in a controlled way.

Functions of the Spine

The spine is designed to do four things simultaneously: 1) to protect the spinal cord that serves as the primary communication conduit between your brain and the rest of your body; 2) to serve as a structural support and attachment for muscles and ligaments; 3) to provide the mobility and flexibility to allow you to bend forward to touch your toes, swim, throw a baseball, and turn your head; and 4) the spine is responsible for transmitting body weight when walking and standing.

Unfortunately, with this degree of mobility and flexibility comes potential instability and susceptibility to injury.

Protection

Your spinal cord is a very soft and delicate bundle of nerves linking the communication between the brain and the rest of the body. Any damage to the spinal cord can result in devastating disabilities. One of the important roles of the spine is to encase the spinal cord in a strong bony structure for protection.

Structure

When viewed from the front or back, the spine should appear perfectly straight and symmetrical, reflecting the fact that your body is also symmetrical when viewed from the front or back. When viewed from the side, however, four major curves should be seen – one in each of the cervical, thoracic, lumbar, and sacral regions. In both the cervical and lumbar regions of the spine, the curves bend backward. These are called "lordotic" curves. The curves in the thoracic and sacral regions bend forward. These are called "kyphotic" curves. As strange as it may seem, these curves actually add a considerable amount of strength and resiliency to the spine. Think about the curves as being like a spring, allowing the spine to flex and

Spinal Innervation Chart

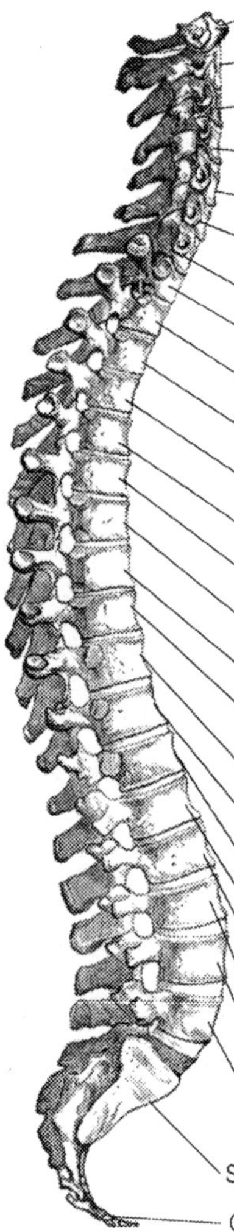

The Negative Effects of a Subluxation

C1	Headaches, nervousness, insomnia, dizziness, hypertension, amnesia.
C2	Allergies, earache, sinus and eye problems, deafness.
C3	Neuralgia, neuritis, acne, eczema.
C4	Hay fever, adenoid infections, post nasal drip.
C5	Laryngitis, hoarseness, sore throat.
C6	Stiff neck, upper arm pain, tonsilitis, croup, whooping cough.
C7	Bursitis, colds, thyroid conditions, goiter, tennis elbow.
T1	Asthma, cough, shortness of breath, lower arm and hand pain.
T2	Functional heart conditions and certain chest pains.
T3	Bronchitis, pleurisy, pneumonia, chest congestion.
T4	Gall bladder problems, jaundice, shingles.
T5	Liver conditions, fevers, low blood pressure, anemia, arthritis.
T6	Indigestion, gastric reflux.
T7	Diabetes, stomach ulcers, gastritis, hypoglycemia.
T8	Hiccoughs, decreased immune function.
T9	Allergies, hives, hypertension, hypoglycemia, obesity, hair loss.
T10	Kidney problems, chronic fatigue, nephritis.
T11	Acne, eczema, boils,
T12	Rheumatism, intestinal gas,
L1	Constipation, colitis, dysentery, diarrhea.
L2	Appendicitis, cramps, acidosis, varicose veins.
L3	Bladder and menstrual problems, bed wetting, impotency, knee pain.
L4	Sciatica, back pain.
L5	Leg weakness, poor leg circulation.
Sacrum	Scoliosis
Coccyx	Hemmorrhoids, pruritis.

absorb shock much better than if it were straight. When a region of the spine loses its normal curve, the discs that separate the vertebrae can begin to degenerate and joints in that area can become less mobile.

Movement

The spine is not just a rigid support system for the rest of the body. Its design is essential to your ability to walk, run, lift, reach, climb, or perform any other activity. To allow this great degree of movement, the spine must be very flexible. However, this flexibility comes with an increased risk of injury. This is why the areas of the spine that have the greatest degree of flexibility – the neck and low back – are the most likely to become injured, while the areas with the most stability – the skull, thoracic spine, and the sacrum – are less prone to injury.

A Healthy Spine

To achieve a healthy back, every part of the spine – the bones, joints, discs, ligaments, muscles, and nerves – must all work in unison, each contributing to stability, power, movement, strength, and flexibility. Often, we go about our daily activities without worrying about back pain. But when we suffer from back pain, we are reminded of just how important a healthy spine is to our quality of life. With the right treatment and regular care, our spines can remain strong and healthy throughout our lives.

2

Low Back Pain

"Nobody in America should be allowed to have back surgery unless they have seen a chiropractor first."

- Robert Mendelsohn, M.D.

Low back pain is very common in the United States. In fact, eighty percent of all people suffer from back pain at some point in their lives. Back pain is the second most common reason for visits to the doctor's office, outnumbered only by upper-respiratory infections. It has been estimated that low back pain affects more than half of the adult population each year, and more than 10% of all people experience frequent bouts of low back pain.

The susceptibility of the low back to injury and pain is due to the fact that the low back, like the neck, is a very unstable part of the spine, unlike the thoracic spine, which is supported and stabilized by the rib cage. This instability allows us to have a great deal of mobility, but it comes at the cost of increased risk of injury.

As long as it is healthy and functioning correctly, the low back can withstand tremendous forces without injury. Professional powerlifters can pick up several hundred pounds off the floor without injuring their low back. However, if the low back is not moving properly or has weakened supporting muscles, something as simple as taking a bag of groceries out of the trunk of the car, picking something up off the floor, or even simply bending down to pet the cat can cause a low back injury.

Until recently, researchers believed that back pain would heal on its own. We have learned, however, that this is not always true. Recent studies showed that when back pain is left untreated, it may go away temporarily but will most likely return. For this reason, it is important to seek care with a qualified practitioner when back or neck pain occurs or when you experience an injury. Chiropractors who focus on early intervention, treatment, and education to prevent recurrence often successfully manage low back problems before they become chronic.

Patient Education is Critical

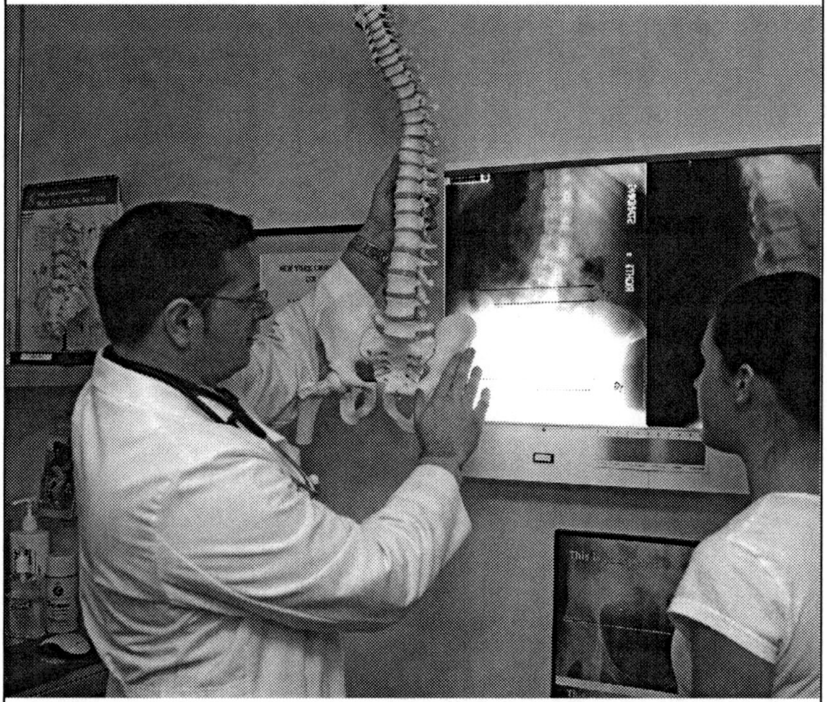

Your doctor should always take the time to explain what is wrong and your options for treatment. He should also take the time to answer any questions or concerns you may have. An educated patient is a healthy patient.

The Causes of Low Back Pain

As we talked about earlier, the back is a complicated structure of bones, joints, discs, ligaments, and muscles. You can sprain ligaments, strain muscles, rupture disks, develop trigger points, and irritate joints, all of which can lead to back

Anatomy of the Low Back

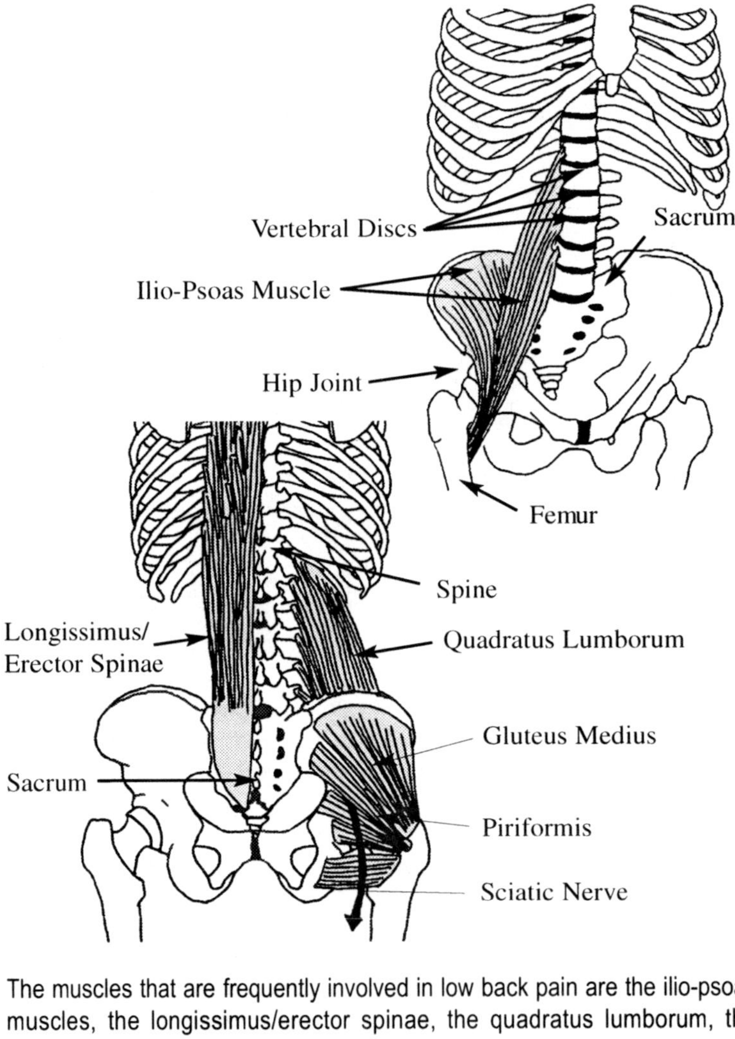

The muscles that are frequently involved in low back pain are the ilio-psoas muscles, the longissimus/erector spinae, the quadratus lumborum, the gluteus muscles, and piriformis muscles of the hip. Weak abdominal muscles can also lead to low back instability and pain.

pain. While sports injuries or accidents can lead to injury and pain, sometimes even the simplest movements, like picking up a pencil from the floor, can have painful results. In addition, conditions such as arthritis, poor posture, obesity, psychological stress, kidney stones, kidney infections, blood clots, tumors, or bone loss can also lead to low back pain.

Due to the fact that there so many things that can cause low back pain, and some of those things can be quite serious if left untreated, it is important to seek professional help. Chiropractors are experts at diagnosing the cause and determining the proper treatment for low back pain. In this next section we will address the most common causes of back pain.

The Intervertebral Disc

As we previously discussed, the intervertebral disc is a spongy pad that separates the vertebrae of the spine, creating a shock-absorbing cushion. Most experts agree that the disc is one of the most common sources of back pain. The center of the disc, called the nucleus, is made of a gel-like material. This nucleus is surrounded by annular fibers that encircle and contain the nucleus. These fibers are arranged much like a series of rubber bands and are designed to contain the nucleus.

Disc Herniation

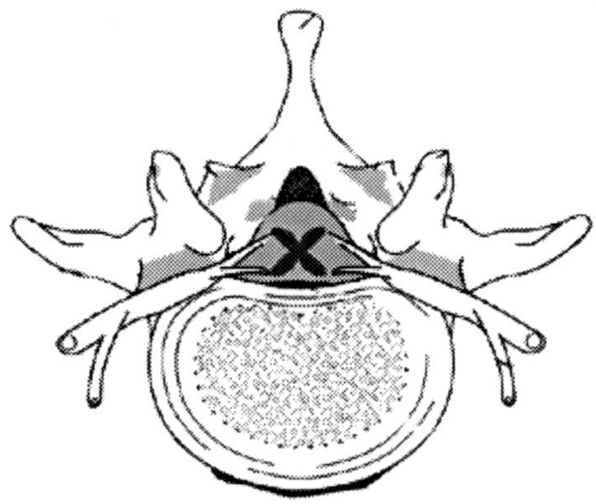

Normal Disc

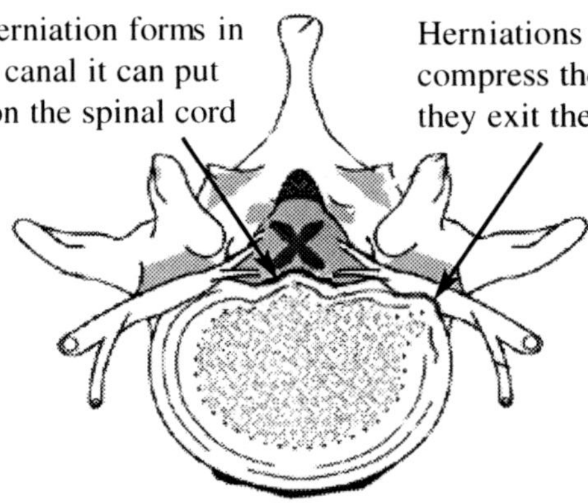

Herniated Disc

Fortunately, not all disc herniations cause pain. But when the herniation puts pressure on either the spinal cord or the individual nerve roots as they exit the spine, the resulting pain can be quite severe and usually radiates into other parts of the body, such as down one or both legs.

Degenerative Disc Disease

Beginning in our teens, the intervertebral disc begins to lose some of its fluid. During this dehydration process, the disc is receiving less nutrition, slowly causing the disc to lose its ability to resist compression; and the space where the disc lies begins to lose its height.

When the space begins to narrow due to a loss of fluid within the disc, problems can occur. Degenerative disc disease is the term used by health care providers to describe this process. On an x-ray, this often shows up as a loss of the normal space between vertebrae. More specific tests, such as an MRI, may show a loss of water content and dehydration, narrowing of the holes where the spinal nerves exit (known as foramen), and ripping of the layers of cartilage (called annular tears) in the outer portion of the disc. Although these findings can be seen with people without any symptoms, the loss of disc space and fluid, and the associated pathology, can cause significant pain and disability.

Disc Injuries

When the nucleus of an intervertebral disc loses its fluid, the normal motion of the spine at that level is lost. The resulting abnormality can cause tearing or ripping of the outer portion of the disc. This may result in a series of events that allow the nucleus to push its way through the outer annulus, putting pressure on the spinal nerve roots. This essentially "chokes" the nerve and often results in severe pain, burning, or numbness in the low back, buttocks, or legs.

Often, it is difficult for the person with disc problems to sit for very long, as this increases the pressure within the disc. Standing, too, may be difficult, and when a person with a severe disc problem stands up, they often cannot straighten into a full erect standing position. Many times, they lean to one side or another, which is the body's way of protecting the nerve from being compressed further.

A bulging, protruded, or slipped disc occurs when the inner nucleus pushes on the outer annular fibers of the disc, pressing on spinal nerves.

A ruptured or herniated disc occurs when the nucleus pushes through the outer fibers of the disc and leaks into the spinal foramen or canal, irritating the spinal nerves by direct pressure or an inflammatory reaction. Leg pain, numbness, burning, or weakness is often the unfortunate result.

Although disc problems may be diagnosed by history and physical examination, an MRI scan best shows disc disorders and will confirm the diagnosis.

Despite the severity of pain often associated with a disc disorder, most cases of disc problems respond very well to conservative chiropractic treatments. Chiropractic manipulation is often useful in relieving the pain, reducing disc protrusion, and restoring movement to irritated or inflamed joints that surround disc problems.

Flexion-distraction disc decompression therapy has been shown to be effective in cases of bulging and herniated discs. This technique, which is discussed later in Chapter 7, is aimed at decreasing pressure within the disc. Exercises from your chiropractor, such as Williams Flexion or McKenzie Method, may help reduce pain and allow for rehabilitation of the region.

In about 2% of disc cases, surgery will be necessary to remove the disc or decompress the area where the nerve exits.

Facet Syndrome

Facet joint disorders are some of the most common of all the recurrent spinal problems. The spinal facet joints are found at every spinal level and provide about 20% of the torsional (twisting) motion and stability in the back. These joints stabilize the spine while allowing for flexibility and protection of the spinal nerves. Each facet joint is positioned in the spine at a specific angle to provide the needed limits and ease of motion as to prevent slippage of one vertebra over another.

Facet joints are in almost perpetual motion. Because of this, these spinal joints may wear out or become degenerated. This process is not age-related and can occur to anyone at any time. When the facet joints become worn down, the cartilage within them may become thin or disappear, resulting in pain and decreased motion.

Each facet joint is coated by a very low friction moist cartilage and is surrounded by a capsule that has a rich supply of nerves, as well as a sticky fluid lubricant for the joint. This fluid, known as synovial fluid, may become less viscous and turn from an egg white consistency to that of chicken fat. Small pieces of joint cartilage, called synovial tags or meniscoids, may become trapped within the joint, causing severe pain with certain movements. This sets the stage for pain, limited motion, and interference with normal daily activities.

Symptoms of facet joint problems are often unpredictable. Usually, there are several episodes over a period of time. In many cases, pain may be very localized over the involved joint. It is rare that a facet injury causes pain or numbness in the leg, but the pain can radiate into the buttocks, groin, and thigh. In an attempt to protect the injury, muscles often go into spasm around the joint. This spasm will often be painful as well (see "Sprains, Strains, and Spasm" section). Typically, facet syndrome pain will become worse when a person bends backwards or rotates to one side.

Although common, facet syndrome is not always easy to diagnose, and several other problems (abdominal tumors, spinal fractures, kidney stones, etc.) need to be ruled out by your doctor before the diagnosis is confirmed. Chiropractors are well trained in the process of differentially diagnosing this problem through not only physical examination, but other tests such as x-rays, blood-work, or urinalysis when necessary to exclude serious pathology. Although well trained in hands-on diagnosis, therapists (massage therapists, physical therapists, occupational therapists, etc.), do not have the training or ability to order tests which may help them confirm what they think is wrong.

Fortunately, facet syndrome can often be effectively managed without surgery or the prolonged use of drugs. Chiropractic manipulation is the treatment that has been most prescribed for pain that is coming from the facet joints. Spinal manipulation, combined with exercise, often helps individuals gain relief and prevent or minimize recurrences of facet syndrome.

In addition to traditional chiropractic treatment, manipulation under joint anesthesia (MUJA) is a new procedure that has promising results in achieving longer-term benefit than traditional treatment. I have had the opportunity to perform this procedure with great success. MUJA is discussed in more depth later in this book.

Vertebral Subluxation Complex

The Vertebral Subluxation Complex, or VSC, is a group of symptoms that can arise when one vertebra has lost its normal position in relation to the one above or below it. The VSC can be seen anywhere in the spinal column and can be responsible for dysfunction in the low back, mid-back, or neck. Put simply, a subluxation is a disruption in the normal movement of a spinal segment that can result in pain, inflammation, nerve irritation, and loss of normal function.

I often refer to the VSC as a "low-grade facet syndrome." Before a spinal problem becomes advanced, and sometimes before symptoms even occur, slight distortions, malrotations, or misalignments of the spine can occur secondary to poor posture, scoliosis or congenital disorders, injury, muscular incoordination, or early spinal degenerative disc or joint disease. With trauma or advanced arthritis, the VSC can become more insidious and painful.

Chiropractors are the only professionals who are trained to diagnose and treat what are called spinal subluxations. The word *subluxation* comes from the Latin words meaning "to dislocate" (luxare) and "somewhat" or "slightly" (sub). So the term *vertebral subluxation* literally means "a slight dislocation (misalignment) of the bones in the spine."

Although this term was adequate in the 1800s when much was still misunderstood about the human body, today the word "subluxation" has changed in meaning to capture the complex neurological, structural, and functional changes that occur when a spinal joint is not moving properly. For this reason, chiropractors usually refer to a subluxation of the spine as a "Vertebral Subluxation Complex" or "VSC" for short. There are actually five components that contribute to the Vertebral Subluxation Complex (VSC).

1) Spinal Kinesiopathology. This is the "bone and joint" component of the VSC and is seen when a vertebra is out of position, not moving properly, or has undergone degeneration.

Physical injury, emotional stress, or other trauma may also cause this problem. With altered joint mechanics, there is loss of normal bending, turning, or other movements.

2) Neuropathophysiology. When spinal biomechanics are altered, there is a disruption of the normal messages traveling along the nerve fibers, which are often pinched, twisted, choked, stretched, distorted, or otherwise irritated by abnormal spinal function.

This may result in numbness, tingling, or pain in the area of dysfunction or anywhere along the course of the irritated nerve. The result can be distorted signals from the brain to the nerve's target area, and subsequent dysfunction.

3) Myopathology. Since nerves exiting the spine control the muscles that help stabilize the vertebrae, the muscular component is an integral part of the Vertebral Subluxation Complex.

When there is abnormal spinal movement, certain spinal support muscles may weaken or atrophy. Other muscles around the subluxation may go into spasm to protect the injured or dysfunctional spinal segment. A vicious cycle ensues, as muscle spasm pulls the vertebrae further out of normal position. Spinal muscular support will be difficult or impossible as muscular tissue becomes fibrotic and produces scar tissue or when it becomes weak and atrophies (shrinks). Lack of muscular coordination can contribute to bulging or herniated discs, which may place pressure on nerve roots or the spinal cord itself.

4) Histopathology. The VSC can also effect the tendons, ligaments, and other soft tissues surrounding the spine. Swelling and inflammation can cause these soft tissues to become painful or easily torn, stretched, or scarred, leaving the spine with instability or restriction. Spinal instability from poor ligament strength can contribute to early attempts by the body to stabilize the vertebral segment by depositing calcium, which can seen as bony spurs on an x-ray.

5) Pathophysiology. Poorly functioning spinal joints often change the local chemistry in that area of the spine. As early as 1969, studies have repeatedly shown inflammatory chemicals such as phospholipase A2, as well as an acidic pH, to be present in spinal nerves. When these chemicals are released, they can cause chemical inflammation and irritation of the tissues and nerves in that region of the spine, as well as into the areas where the inflamed nerve extends.

These changes may get progressively worse over time if they are not treated correctly, leading to chronic pain, inflammation, arthritis, muscle trigger points, the formation of bone spurs, loss of movement, as well as muscle weakness and spasm. Chiropractors have known the dangers of the Vertebral Subluxation Complex ever since the birth of the profession. More and more, scientific research is demonstrating the impact that subluxations have on the various tissues of the body.

In order to be truly healthy, it is vital for your nervous system to be functioning free of interference from subluxations. Spinal subluxations can often be detected by feeling the area (known as palpation), reading x-rays, or doing a postural analysis or surface EMG. Chiropractors are the only health professionals trained in the detection, location, and correction of the Vertebral Subluxation Complex.

Sciatica

Sciatica is not a cause of low back pain, but is a non-specific term referring to pain, burning, or numbness in the buttock or leg.

The sciatic nerve is the largest nerve in the body. This nerve exits the spine and runs through your hip area and buttocks and down each leg. The sciatic nerve then branches into smaller nerves as it travels down the leg, providing feeling to your thighs and legs. It also controls the muscles in your legs and feet.

Sciatica is a sign that there is an underlying problem putting pressure on the nerve. The nerve can be pinched, mechanically compressed, or inflamed anywhere along its course from the spine to the toes. Sciatica is seen in all age groups but is most common in people between the ages of 30 and 50.

Most commonly, the sciatic nerve is compressed by a disc problem (bulges, protrusions, or herniations of disc material) in your lower back. These cases often resolve with non-surgical treatments such as chiropractic adjustments, physiotherapy modalities, disc traction/decompression techniques, and home exercises. Sometimes, injections of medication near the nerve will decrease the inflammation associated with sciatic pain.

In very rare cases of sciatic nerve compression with a serious condition known as cauda equina syndrome, the legs may become progressively weak, and bowel or bladder incontinence can occur. This is a medical emergency and usually requires immediate medical attention and probably surgery.

Piriformis Syndrome or "pseudosciatica" is a condition that occurs when the sciatic nerve is compressed as it runs through the piriformis muscle, which is located in the buttock area. As this is a muscular problem, surgery is never prescribed for this syndrome. Often, a short course of chiropractic care and home stretches will minimize the pain associated with piriformis syndrome.

Spinal Stenosis

Stenosis is a term used by health professionals to describe a narrowing of any opening or hole within the body. You may have heard of arterial stenosis, a condition where the arteries that carry blood away from the heart are blocked or narrowed by plaques or fatty deposits.

As the term implies, spinal stenosis is a narrowing of the spinal foramen or canal that results in compression of the nerves that exit the spine to control the body. Just as a narrowed artery will not give adequate blood supply to the organ it transports blood to, a narrowed spinal canal or nerve opening can result in pain, weakness, or poor neural supply to its target body parts.

There are two types of spinal stenosis: foraminal stenosis and canal stenosis. Foraminal stenosis is a narrowing of the small foramen, or hole, that a single spinal nerve passes through after it exits the safety of the bony spinal canal. This compression, which is often due to bulging discs, bony spurs, vertebral subluxation, or facet joint arthritis or growth, is usually associated with pain, burning, or numbness along the route of one spinal nerve. A doctor who is well trained in diagnosis is often able to localize the nerve involved by checking the patient's sensation along specific nerve root paths or tapping specific reflexes.

Spinal stenosis, on the other hand, is a more "generalized" narrowing. With spinal stenosis, the entire spinal opening for the spinal cord (called the spinal canal) is decreased. The causes of spinal stenosis are the same as those seen with foraminal stenosis, but because the entire spinal cord (and not one specific nerve) is compressed, symptoms are often felt in both legs. In many cases of spinal stenosis, patients feel better when they bend forward (which has been shown to increase the diameter of the spinal canal), and feel worse after a long walk or when they bend backwards (as this often narrows the space available for the spinal cord within the canal).

Degenerative Joint Disease

Degenerative Joint Disease is sometimes known as "spinal arthritis" or "spondylosis." Many of my patients who have already had x-rays or an MRI tell me that they have "arthritis" in their spine. Although arthritis is common, it is not a diagnosis in and of itself. Instead, spinal arthritis is something to be seen on an x-ray, indicating that there is a problem. It often shows up as claw-like bony spurs, loss of space between vertebrae, poor alignment of one vertebra in relation to another, or narrowing of the foramen where the nerve exits.

Spinal arthritis is a sign of dysfunction and can be prevented. It is not inevitable and is not age-related. I have seen hundreds of elderly patients with no signs of degenerative changes on their x-rays, and I have encountered just as many 30-year olds with advanced changes on theirs.

The cascade of events that cause spinal arthritis has been well documented by the eminent Drs. Kirkaldy and Willis, as well as Dr. Panjabi. It has become accepted in the medical community that the formation of bony spurs in the spine is in fact a response to abnormal motion or dysfunction in a spinal joint. These spurs, which until recently were written off as "arthritis," are actually a sign that the body, in its infinite wisdom, is attempting to stabilize a dysfunctional joint by the only way it can - through the laying down of calcium.

As with most spinal disorders, chiropractic care is effective in the treatment of degenerative joint disease. By restoring and maintaining movement to the spinal joints through chiropractic manipulation, the physical effects (loss of motion, stiffness, etc.) to those with spinal arthritis may be kept to a minimum or prevented altogether. Rehabilitation and home exercises prescribed by your chiropractor will help keep the stabilizing spinal muscles strong and flexible to prevent further problems. In many cases, nutritional advice or dietary considerations may be helpful.

Leg Length Inequality "Short Leg Syndrome"

Having one leg shorter than another is like driving a car with two different tires. Low back, hip, knee, or leg pain can be caused by such a disorder, which may go undetected for years. Leg length inequality is often discovered by a variety of means used by chiropractors, orthopedic surgeons, and other health care providers. These include x-rays, measurements on a patient with a tape measure, or more advanced tests such as a scintogram.

A 1983 study published in *Spine* showed that only 43.5% of a control group had more than a 5mm leg length discrepancy, whereas over 75% of people with chronic low back pain have one leg shorter than the other. Leg length inequality has the potential to cause problems over time through altered spinal biomechanics and abnormal weight bearing. This, in turn, can contribute to the potential for injury and a prolonged recovery when other spinal problems exist.

Pre-existing or co-existing spinal problems such as leg length inequality, poor muscle tone, vertebral subluxations, or degenerative conditions often "set the stage" for spinal problems in the future.

In some cases, however, this problem is not the only reason for back pain and may have no significance whatsoever. For example, a small leg length discrepancy in an accountant with back pain while sitting at his desk is less of a concern than a large leg length difference in a marathon runner who experiences back pain while running. As a holistic practitioner, a qualified chiropractor will be able to look at the "big picture" and diagnose whether or not this structural problem has any effect on your current health status or problem. If he or she thinks that the inequality is an issue, foot orthotics or a heel lift may be prescribed along with a course of chiropractic adjustments and exercises to normalize spinal biomechanics.

The fact that muscular and structural distortions contribute to back problems is not lost on the medical profession. For example, in a 1996 article in *Spine*, Gordon Waddell, M.D. aptly pointed out that when disc herniations occur, they are often superimposed upon existing conditions such as dysfunction, degeneration, and deconditioning.

Spondylolisthesis

Spondylolisthesis is a condition that results from a fracture in an area of the vertebrae that allows that vertebra to slip forward upon the one below it. These fractures can be the result of wear and tear or trauma such as a bad fall or sports injury. More often, however, this slippage is the result of a stress fracture due to repeated stress on a weak area of the spine. This is often seen in young athletes such as football or hockey players, gymnasts, or dancers. It can also be found in older individuals as a result of degenerative weakening of this region of the spine.

In some cases, x-rays will reveal that this slippage is excessive, causing the spine to be unstable. Because there is potential for the unstable vertebrae to slip and cause neurological damage, surgery is often required to stabilize the area.

Patients with a stable spondylolisthesis often respond extremely well to chiropractic care. Chiropractic manipulation of dysfunctional spinal joints (usually the joints above or below the slippage) in patients with spondylolisthesis is often as effective as it is with patients without the disorder.

Flexion Distraction technique has also been shown to be effective for this problem, especially if the repeated slippage has caused disc damage and narrowing of the area in between the affected vertebrae. Restriction of certain activities and the use of a brace may also be helpful.

Specific exercises to strengthen and stabilize the region are extremely useful in these cases, but certain exercises should be avoided. A properly trained Doctor of Chiropractic will help you choose the appropriate exercise program for this unique spinal disorder.

Sacroiliac Syndrome

The sacroiliac joint (SI joint) consists of the sacrum (the triangle-shaped bone at the base of the spine) and the ilium (pelvic bone). This joint is the connection between the ground and your spine. It acts as a shock absorber, transmitting all the forces of the upper body to the hips, pelvis, and legs.

Dysfunction in the sacroiliac joint is thought to cause low back and occasionally leg pain. Sometimes, the pain is similar to that of a herniated lumbar disc or facet joint disorder.

Treatment of pain emanating from the sacroiliac joint is based on an accurate diagnosis because the SI joint may become painful for two completely different reasons: (1) The joint may not be moving or mobile. This is known as a hypomobility, fixation, or sacroiliac subluxation. This type of pain is often felt on one side of the low back, buttocks, groin, or leg just above the knee. (2) The SI joint has the potential to move too much. This is referred to as hypermobility or instability.

In my office, hypermobile sacroiliac joints are often seen in pregnant patients with low back pain. Often, they are referred to me by their OB/GYN for natural and safe treatment. Because of hormonal effects on the sacroiliac ligaments that cause the relaxation of the pelvis for the birthing process, the SI joint can become too "loose." These ligaments, which "hold" the pelvic bones together, can become over-relaxed, causing the muscles of the pelvis, abdomen, low back, and hips to compensate, resulting in pain and spasm. These sacroiliac ligaments can also be torn by a traumatic event such as a fall, accident, or lifting injury.

To make treatment more challenging, it is often the cause of SI joint pain that must be corrected before any long-term relief is obtained. Many patients in my clinic have undergone multiple treatments and sometimes unnecessary surgery, for what turns out to be an SI joint disorder.

Chiropractic care has been the treatment of choice for Sacroiliac Syndrome for decades. Traditional physio-therapy (heat, ultrasound, etc.) has been shown to have mild effects on the healing process of SI syndromes. Braces and support belts may be used to temporarily stabilize the joint and allow the ligaments to heal (which can also be facilitated by nutritional support). However, prolonged bracing may weaken the muscles around the joint, so a transition to a supervised program of chiropractic manipulation and exercise is imperative.

In many cases, abnormal biomechanics must be corrected before the SI joint dysfunction stabilizes. This is often done through Foot Leveler orthotics (which can correct leg length inequality, excessive turning (torsion) of the feet, knees, or hips), heel lifts, or neuromuscular re-education training with a qualified chiropractic practitioner.

Failed Back Surgery Syndrome

When conditions are commonly seen in a health care setting, they are assigned an ICD (International Classification of Disease) code for use by doctors in notifying insurance companies of an accepted diagnosis on the bill. The ICD code for a failed back surgery is 722.83. There is no ICD code for failed knee surgery syndrome, failed cardiac surgery syndrome, or failed rotator cuff surgery syndrome. In 2001, *The New England Journal of Medicine* reported that surgery is overused in the treatment of back pain. (*NEJM*; 2001:344(5) pp363-69).

Even with the best surgeons and for the best surgical indications (reasons), spinal surgery is no more than 95% successful. This means that no less than 5 out of every 100 patients who undergo spinal surgery will still have back pain afterwards.

Spinal surgery is not performed to literally "cut out" the patient's pain. It is an attempt to change anatomy and remove or change whatever tissue is the probable cause of the patient's pain.

Spinal surgery is only basically able to accomplish two things: (1) decompress a nerve that is being pinched or choked, or (2) stabilize a painful spinal joint.

There are reasons for spinal surgery, which we will discuss in Chapter 9. Certain spinal surgeries, such as microdiscectomy and spinal fusion, have a more favorable outcome than others. The key, however, is to make sure that a patient has exhausted all conservative options for care, and that the area to be operated on is, in fact, the pain-producing tissue. This is well beyond the scope of this book and may require diagnostic injections or discography (see Chapter 9).

There are several causes of failed back surgery syndrome. Unfortunately, spinal fusion procedures have the potential to transfer motion to the level above the operation, which may speed up the degenerative process at that level and result in pain.

Lumbar decompression surgeries may result in recurrent disc herniation (which is seen in 5-10% of cases), inadequate decompression, or nerve damage that either occurs during surgery or does not heal after decompression. Sometimes, decompressing a nerve during surgery may temporarily inflame the nerve and result in pain until the inflammation subsides. Scar tissue may form around the nerve after surgery.

In general, if there has not been improvement in 3 months after a spinal surgery, the operation may be deemed unsuccessful; further diagnostic tests or treatment may be reasonable.

Of course, there are technical problems with spinal surgery as well. Operating on the wrong spinal level or "missing" the disc or bone that is pinching the nerve is possible. Fortunately, these complications are very uncommon. Spine surgeons are extremely well trained. They often consider surgery to be a last resort and usually make every attempt to pinpoint what is causing the patient's pain.

Treatment of Failed Back Surgery Syndrome is based on what part of the spine is causing the pain. Many chiropractors are trained in the treatment of Failed Back Surgery Syndrome. These are often complicated cases and usually require a structured treatment program.

Stretching can help reduce scar tissue formation if it is done within 6 to 12 weeks after the surgery. Education on proper posture, body position, and movement is often helpful. Range of motion, strengthening, and exercise programs definitely have a role. In cases where another disc is causing pain, decompression therapy or epidural injections may provide some relief. When the sacroiliac or facet joints are painful, gentle chiropractic manipulation, facet injections, or the MUJA procedure may reduce symptoms and increase mobility. If the pain is coming from irritated or tight muscles or trigger points, soft tissue therapies have the potential to minimize the associated pain.

Sprains, Strains, and Spasm

Muscle pain is only thought to be the cause of 20% of all back pain. In most cases where there has been trauma or injury, the muscles around a degenerated, dysfunctional, or inflamed area of the spine are in spasm or tighten in an attempt to protect the area. In cases of direct trauma such as falls, car accidents, or sports injuries, there may be extensive damage to the soft tissues. When a tendon or muscle has been injured, it is called a "strain." If a ligament is injured, torn, or damaged, it is referred to as a "sprain." In most cases of spinal soft tissue injury, both the tendons and ligaments are involved. This is referred to as a "sprain-strain."

The role of chiropractic care in managing sprain-strain injuries to the muscles, tendons, and ligaments is based on relieving pain, promoting full tissue healing, restoration of function, reduction of the potential for re-injury, and prevention of accelerated spinal degeneration.

When an injury to the back or neck occurs, there are four phases of healing that the region must undergo. Qualified Doctors of Chiropractic have been extensively trained in specific treatment procedures and goals specific to each phase of healing.

Phase 1: Active Swelling

Within the first 12-72 hours of an injury, swelling occurs as cells enter the area to prevent further damage. This often results in pain and loss of motion in that area. During this phase, your chiropractor will recommend rest and support of the area by taping, bracing, or other protective means. Ice is often used during this period to reduce pain and to minimize spasm and swelling.

Phase 2: Passive Congestion

The second phase of healing an injury is known as that of "passive congestion." This usually begins in the second to fourth day, and during this time the fluid in the injured area tends to become counterproductive, causing increased pain and loss of motion. Doctors of Chiropractic often use manipulation or mobilization during this phase to slowly restore movement to the region, resulting in pain relief and increased motion. Physiotherapy modalities and basic exercises may also reduce unnecessary congestion.

Phase 3: Repair

Around the fifth day after an injury, scar tissue begins to form around the area. This is known as the repair phase and can continue for up to 6 weeks. Lack of motion during this phase of healing can be detrimental, and scar tissue may form excessively, resulting in stiffness, limited range of motion, and poor joint mechanics. If motion is restored and maintained during this phase, tissues will heal more functionally.

Chiropractic care should continue throughout the repair phase as chiropractic treatment can be effective in restoring motion and proper biomechanics, improving connective tissue alignment, preventing scar tissue shortening, and restoring normal muscular tone and coordination.

Phase 4: Remodeling

The final stage of injury healing is known as the remodeling phase. This phase can take 3-14 weeks and sometimes up to a year to complete. During this time, connective tissue remodels to provide strength and flexibility around the area of injury. Chiropractic treatment continues to be useful during this final phase, as it assists in the continued improvement of motion and flexibility, maintenance of function, reduction of pain, and minimizing the risk of reinjury.

Osteoporosis

Osteoporosis is a disease that causes bones to be thin and brittle. People with osteoporosis are at greater risk of breaking a hip or a wrist and of having a compression fracture in their spine. In the U.S. today, 10 million individuals already have osteoporosis and 34 million more have low bone mass, placing them at increased risk for this disease. Osteoporosis is more common in women - 50% of women and 25% of men will have an osteoporosis-related fracture in their lifetime.

Osteoporosis results when bone density decreases. This can be due to inadequate calcium or vitamin D intake, excessive calcium loss secondary to disease or medications, and lack of weight bearing exercise. As you get older, your risk of osteoporosis increases. Other risk factors include Caucasian or Southeast Asian ethnicity, small frame size or low body weight, family history, and smoking.

Unfortunately, you may not realize that you have osteoporosis until you break a bone or begin to develop a hump in your back. Osteoporosis will not show up on x-rays until bone loss is extensive. The only way to tell if you have osteoporosis is to have a bone density test, or "densitometry." A bone density test uses low-power x-rays to determine how dense your bones are. The denser your bones, the less likely they are to break.

Stress

Whenever you experience stress, your body responds by increasing your blood pressure and heart rate, flooding your body with stress hormones and tightening up your muscles. When you are constantly stressed, the chronic tension causes your muscles to become sore, weak, and loaded with trigger points and muscle tightness and imbalance often result. This can contribute to the Vertebral Subluxation Complex, resulting in a vicious cycle of pain and spinal dysfunction. If you are constantly under stress and you have low back pain, it is important to do some relaxation exercises, such as deep breathing, as well as to get regular physical exercise.

3

Neck and Upper Back Pain

"In nothing do men approach so nearly to the Gods, as in giving health to men."

- Cicero

While not as common as low back pain, neck pain affects almost everyone at some point in their life. Although most cases of neck pain are not due to severe traumatic injury, the pain can be just as disabling whatever the cause. People do not realize how much they move their neck during the day until they are unable to do so. The degree of flexibility of the neck, coupled with the fact that it has the least amount of muscular stabilization and it has to support and move your 14-16 pound head, means that the neck is very susceptible to injury. You can

Anatomy of the Neck and Upper Back

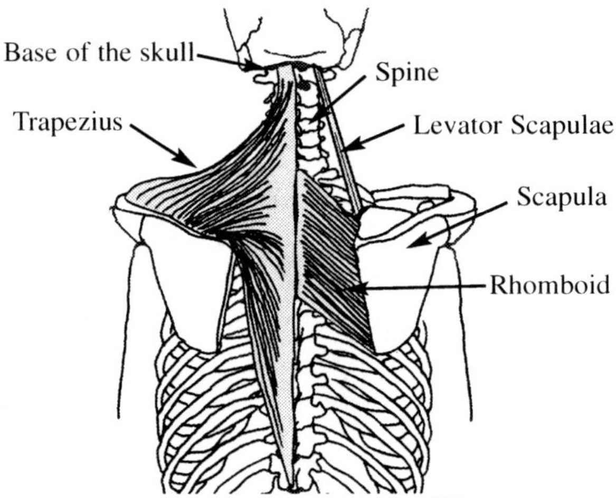

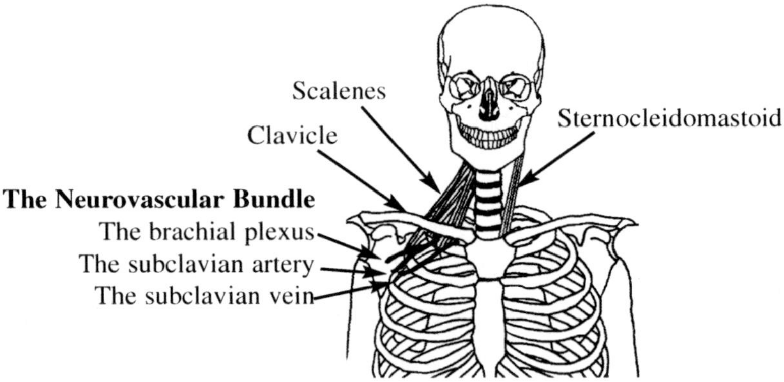

The muscles in the neck and upper back that are most commonly involved with causing pain are the trapezius, rhomboid, levator scapulae, scalenes, and the sternocleidomastoid. The scalenes are particularly problematic due to their proximity to the nerves and blood vessels that feed the arms. Injuries or trigger points in any of these muscles will often lead to pain and loss of function.

picture your neck and head much like a bowling ball being held on top of a stick by small, thin, elastic bands. It doesn't take much force to disrupt that delicate balance.

As you read earlier, the spinal cord runs through a space in the vertebrae to send nerve impulses to every part of the body. Between each pair of cervical vertebrae, the spinal cord sends off large bundles of nerves that run down the arms and to some degree, the upper back. This means that if your arm is hurting, it may actually be a problem in the neck! Symptoms in the arms can include numbness, tingling, cold, aching, and "pins and needles." These symptoms can be confused with carpal tunnel syndrome, a painful condition in the hands that is often found in people who work at computer keyboards or perform other repetitive motion tasks for extended periods.

Problems in the neck can also contribute to headaches, muscle spasms in the shoulders and upper back, ringing in the ears, dizziness and vertigo, temporomandibular joint dysfunction (TMJ), restricted range of motion and chronic muscle tightness in the neck and upper back.

We will talk about the neck and upper back together, because most of the muscles that are associated with the neck either attach to, or are located in, the upper back. These muscles include the trapezius, the levator scapulae, the cervical paraspinal muscles and the scalenes, as well as others.

The Cause of Neck and Upper Back Pain

Most neck and upper back pain is caused by a combination of factors including injury, poor posture, the Vertebral Subluxation Complex, stress, and disc problems.

Traumatic Injuries and Whiplash Syndrome

By far, the most common injury to the neck is a whiplash injury. Whiplash is caused by a sudden movement of the head, either backward, forward, or sideways, that results in the damage to the supporting muscles, ligaments, and other connective tissues in the neck and upper back. Whether from a car accident, sports, or an accident at work, whiplash injuries need to be taken very seriously. Too often people don't seek treatment following a car accident or sports injury because they don't feel pain. Unfortunately, by the time more serious complications develop, some of the damage from the injury may have become permanent. Numerous studies have shown that years after whiplash victims settle their insurance claims, roughly half of them state that they still suffer with symptoms from their injuries.

Injuries to the neck from trauma, such as a motor vehicle accident or sports injury, are common and can be serious.

Because this syndrome is common and often results in chronic pain, I have devoted an entire chapter to understanding whiplash injuries.

Poor Posture

One of the most common causes of neck pain, and sometimes headaches, is poor posture. It's easy to get into bad posture habits without even realizing it - even an activity as "innocent" as reading in bed can ultimately lead to pain, headaches, and more serious problems. The basic rule is simple: keep your neck in a "neutral" position whenever possible. Don't bend or hunch your neck forward for long periods. Also, try not to sit in one position for a long time. If you must sit for an extended period, make sure your posture is good: Keep your head in a neutral position, make sure your back is supported, keep your knees slightly above your hips, and rest your arms if possible. Use a pillow that supports the natural curve of your neck when sleeping.

Poor posture can cause more than neck pain and headaches, however. Poor posture and its effect on overall health was studied in 2005, when a group of medical doctors sought out to determine whether or not there was a correlation between health and a patient's head position as measured by x-rays. This study, published in the September 15th issue of *Spine*, looked at 752 adult patients. These patients were x-rayed from the side, and measurements to determine posture were recorded and correlated with the patient's health status. Findings of this study clearly illustrated that patients with a forward head ("chin-poking") had deterioration of their health status, increased pain, and decreased function.

Because posture is so important, I have devoted an entire section on it in Chapter 10.

Cervical Facet Syndrome

Facet syndrome in the neck is similar to that in the low back, which is discussed in Chapter 2. When facet joints in the neck are locked up or irritated, you may experience a lack of motion, sharp pain when bending your head back or sideways, or a general sense of stiffness in your neck. The pain may also extend into your upper back, shoulders, or upper arm. Facet joint pain rarely extends past the elbow.

According to the October 2005 edition of the *American Journal of Pain Management,* 54-67% of chronic neck pain is caused by facet joints. This article goes on to recommend manipulation, traction, and other treatments commonly used by Doctors of Chiropractic for neck pain.

As with low back facet disorders, chiropractic manipulation often improves motion in the facet joints and helps to restore and maintain motion and flexibility in these joints. Sometimes, the use of a home traction unit may be suggested by your chiropractor. Exercises are often useful in improving function and preventing re-injury.

A 2002 article in *The Annals of Internal Medicine* suggested that manual (hands-on) therapy for neck pain may be more effective than physical therapy or conventional medical care for neck pain. In this study, 183 patients with neck pain were divided into three categories: (1) the first group underwent manual therapy for six weeks, (2) the second group underwent physical therapy, and (3) the third group was given advice on self-care from general practitioners. The results were as follows: 68% of patients who underwent manual therapy were completely recovered versus 50% of those who underwent physical therapy and 36% who received medical care.

Cervical Degenerative Disc Disease

Degenerative disc disease in the neck is similar to that in the low back, which we discussed earlier in Chapter 2. Degenerative disc disease in the cervical spine can be responsible for causing neck pain, headaches, and pain, burning, or numbness in the shoulders and arms.

A 2002 article in *Spine*, which studied 68 patients with degenerative disease of the neck, compared spinal manipulation, rest, and flexion exercises of the neck to surgery. The study concluded that non-surgical care (such as that given by a Doctor of Chiropractic) of neck degeneration is equally as good as surgery.

Cervical spine traction and exercise, two commonly used chiropractic modalities for neck pain, were shown to be more effective than analgesics (pain medications) in a 2002 study published in the *Bangladesh Medical Resource Council Bulletin.*

Cervical Disc Herniation

The discs in your cervical spine can herniate or bulge and put pressure on the nerves that exit from the spine through that area. Although cervical discs do not herniate nearly as often as lumbar discs do, they occasionally can herniate such as when the discs sustain damage from an injury. When this happens, most people experience radiating pain, numbness, tingling, or burning into their upper back, shoulders, arms, hands, and fingers. There have even been some cases of pain that was initially diagnosed as a rotator cuff injury or carpal tunnel syndrome when, in fact, the problem was arising out of herniated or bulging disc in the neck.

Spinal manipulation, when performed by a highly trained Doctor of Chiropractic, can be a safe and effective treatment for cervical disc herniations. However, manipulation alone is often not enough, and is sometimes avoided altogether in these cases, especially in acute (new or severe) cervical disc herniations. Chiropractors use a variety of tests and physical maneuvers on each patient to determine the appropriateness of manipulation.

Chiropractic treatment of disc herniations in the neck is usually coupled with other physical treatments such as a soft

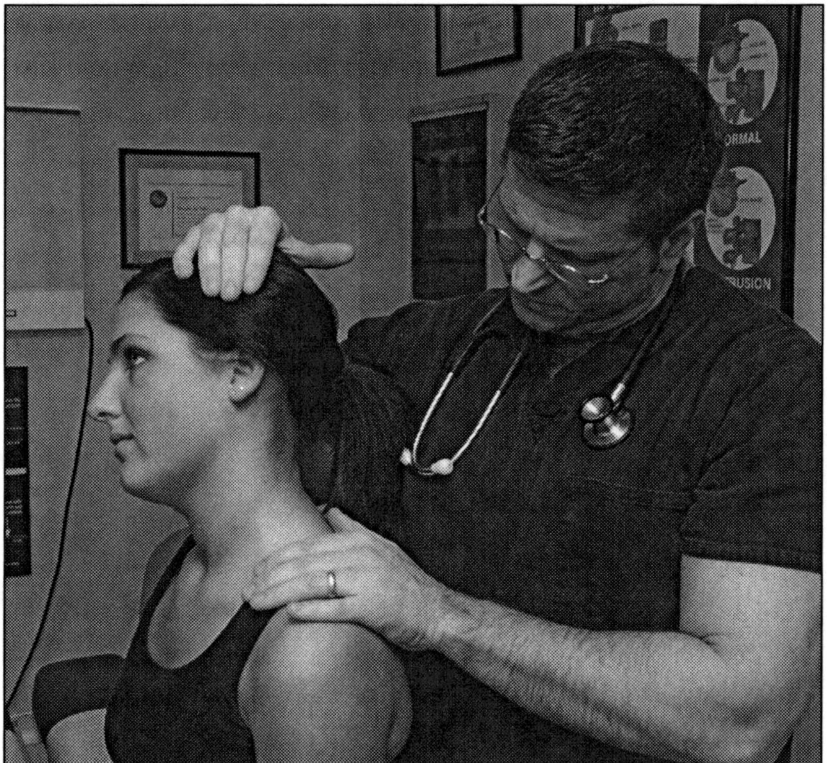

A thorough examination of the neck and upper back by a Doctor of Chiropractic will often reveal the source of your pain.

cervical collar, traction, McKenzie or other exercises protocols, physiotherapy modalities (ultrasound, muscle stimulation), nutritional support, or soft tissue techniques to decrease spasm and pain. These techniques and procedures are discussed further in Chapter 7.

A case series in 1997, published in *The Journal of Manipulative & Physiological Therapeutics*, revealed 80% of disc herniations treated with chiropractic care had a good clinical outcome, and 63% actually had a reduction in size, or complete resolution (this means they disappeared), of the disc herniations seen on the MRI before the study began!

Cervical Vertebral Subluxation Complex

The VSC is discussed in detail in Chapter 2. The VSC is commonly seen at the transitional areas of the spine, such as where the upper neck meets the skull, the middle of the neck (where mechanical stress is greatest), and in the region where the lower neck and upper mid-back meet.

Each of these subluxation areas are associated with particular symptoms. The upper-most subluxations between the cervical spine and the skull tend to cause headaches. The subluxations in the middle of the neck tend to cause neck stiffness and pain. Subluxations at the transition between the cervical and thoracic areas of the spine tend to create chronic muscle tightness and trigger points in the trapezius and levator muscles in the upper back. Subluxations in the middle of the thoracic spine tend to lead to mid-back pain, as well as disease and dysfunction in those areas that receive innervation (nerve supply) from the nerves which exit the thoracic spine.

As we have previously addressed, Doctors of Chiropractic are the only health care providers trained in detecting and treating the Vertebral Subluxation Complex.

Thoracic Outlet Syndrome

Thoracic Outlet Syndrome (TOS) is a group of symptoms caused by compression of blood vessels and nerves in the region where they exit in the lower neck and upper chest area. The nerves and vessels in this area, known as the thoracic outlet, can be compressed by spinal misalignment, skeletal abnormalities, or muscular or postural imbalance.

Care of this problem depends on the site of compression, and usually involves a combination of chiropractic manipulation, manual soft tissue therapies, taping, postural advice and education, exercise to stretch and strengthen surrounding tissues, and other non-surgical treatments.

Cervical Spine Stenosis

Cervical spine stenosis, or narrowing of the spinal canal in the region of the neck, can be caused by disc disorders, degenerative joint changes, or congenital factors. Although seen on an MRI, slight changes in your physical examination, such as changes in your reflexes, may alert your doctor to the problem.

Many patients with this disorder will develop neck pain and arm numbness, similar to that seen in a cervical disc herniation. In more severe cases, there may be a sense of heaviness in the legs or difficulty walking at a brisk pace. Fine motor skills, such as dialing the phone or buttoning up your shirt, may also be affected with this disorder.

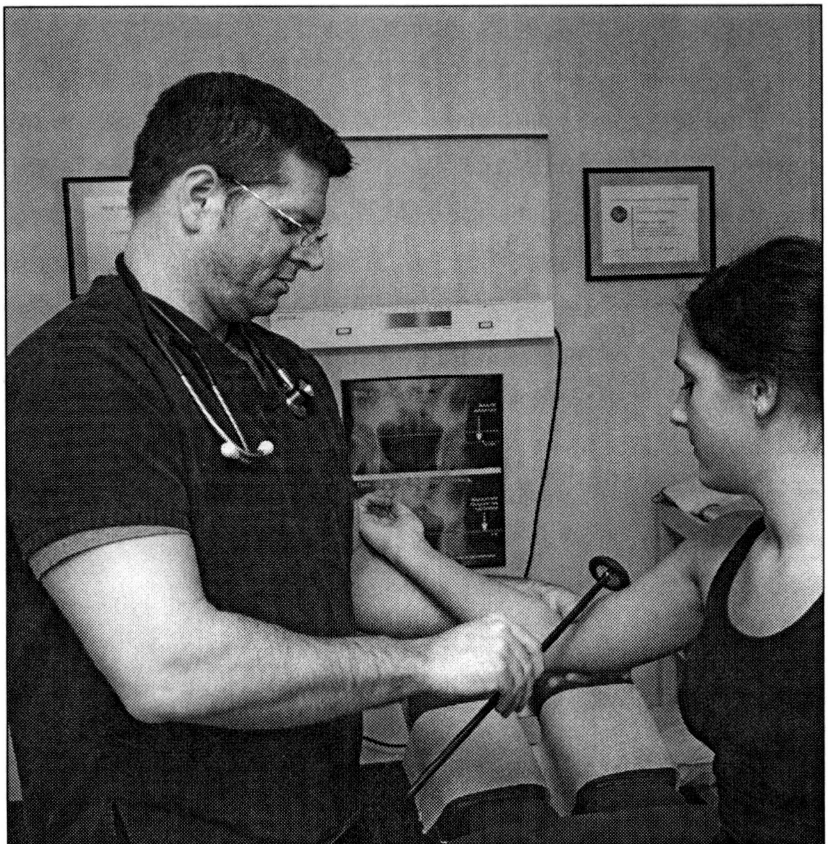

By performing a thorough neurological examination, your doctor may find abnormalities which suggest changes in your spinal cord. Based on these findings, your treatment may be changed, or additional tests or referrals may be suggested to pinpoint the problem before determining the appropriate treatment.

This condition may result in various symptoms, and treatment must be based on the amount of nerve compression and risk for further loss of neurological function. In cases where motor skills are lost or there appears to be compromise of the neurological structures, surgical decompression is necessary.

In early cases of cervical spine stenosis, conservative care may be effective in minimizing symptoms. For example, in a 2002 study published in the *Journal of the Neuromusculoskeletal System*, neck and left shoulder pain in and weakness in a patient with cervical spine stenosis was relieved using Cox Flexion Distraction Cervical Spine Manipulation. Co-treatment between a spinal surgeon and chiropractor is often the best course of action in these cases, as monitoring the condition is often necessary.

Many conditions in the neck cause varying amounts of pain in the neck, head, upper back, shoulders, arms, and hands. A qualified Doctor of Chiropractic has the ability to diagnose your conditions through a thorough physical examination, x-rays, MRI's, or other necessary tests. When a chiropractor arrives at a diagnosis, he or she may treat you or refer you to another health care provider for follow-up care.

Common Causes of Mid-Back Pain

Because there is little motion in the mid-back, many conditions seen in the neck and low back (disc herniations, stenosis, spondylolisthesis, etc.) are rare. However, the mid-back, known as the thoracic spine, is a common area for spinal joint dysfunction due to poor posture, injury, or spinal deformities.

Because of the various organs and tissues located in the thoracic cage, proper diagnosis of a thoracic condition is crucial. Common disorders seen in the mid-back include scoliosis, compression fractures, rib subluxation, thoracic disc herniation, and stress.

Scoliosis

I often see young children with scoliosis. In most cases, they are sent to me after a physical examination at their school creates concern or when a worried parent notices that their child is "crooked." In these young patients, scoliosis should not be painful. The progression of the disease, however, is carefully monitored in young people through periodic examinations and x-rays. If progression is too fast or in a direction that poses danger to internal organs, the curvature must be minimized or prevented through bracing, exercise, and sometimes surgery.

Although their curvature will not increase after they reach maturity, adults with scoliosis have the potential to develop pain due to the uneven wear and tear on spinal facet joints, muscles, ligaments, and discs.

Chiropractic treatment is often effective in treating the symptoms associated with adult scoliosis. Specific spinal adjustments and exercise are usually all that is required to minimize the effects of an abnormal spinal curve. In some cases, gentle traction will relieve nerve pressure caused by "wedging" near the mid-point of the curve.

If an unlevel pelvis or difference in leg length is found, a heel lift or Spinal Pelvic Stabilizer orthotics may help minimize its effects on your spine, normalize abnormal biomechanical stress, and decrease symptoms.

Compression Fractures

When a bone in the spine collapses, it is known as a compression fracture. These fractures are most commonly seen in the thoracic spine and are usually due to conditions such as osteoporosis, a hard fall, or some other type of physical injury.

Doctors of Chiropractic often see patients after a trauma, and can diagnose this problem by ordering x-rays and assessing the level and degree of fracture. CT scans or an MRI may also be useful in making sure that the fracture is stable.

An accurate and early diagnosis of compression fractures may help determine the correct treatment. In many cases, gentle conservative chiropractic treatment and advice from a chiropractor often helps patients deal with their pain and regain function. Therapeutic modalities (electric muscle stimulation, TENs units, heat, etc.) and soft tissue techniques, such as strain-counterstrain, may decrease muscular pain and spasm. Chiropractic manipulation is not recommended for treating this disorder, for obvious reasons.

Patients with compression fractures tend to have osteoporosis, and manual spinal techniques must be modified or avoided altogether. Bracing is another common form of treatment for some types of vertebral compression fractures. Your chiropractor or orthopedic surgeon may recommend a brace to minimize the pressure on the healing vertebral body and prevent further collapse of the bone.

In my office, I stress prevention of compression fractures through adequate dietary intake of calcium and an active lifestyle that includes regular walking, breathing exercises, and weight-bearing exercise and resistance training when appropriate.

Compression fractures will often require the expertise of an orthopedic surgeon, and an integrated "team approach" between your surgeon and chiropractor is often the best course of action. Over the past several years, surgical techniques such as vertebroplasty, as well as other procedures, have allowed the effects of compression fractures to be minimized.

Rib Subluxation "Slipped Rib Syndrome"

A slipped rib, or rib subluxation, is a common cause of mid-back or chest pain. It is seen in people with sharp rib cage pain with deep or heavy breathing. It can often be confused with rib fractures, pleurisy, or disorders of the stomach, esophagus, or heart. These other, more serious conditions, must often be ruled out by your doctor before the diagnosis of rib subluxation is confirmed.

This problem usually arises from trauma to the rib cage or heavy exertion involving the chest wall. It is seen equally in men and women, and results from injury or trauma to the cartilage that attaches to ribs. When these ligaments are injured, the tip of the rib may slip and irritate or pinch the intercostal nerve, causing pain with such movements as twisting, bending, deep breathing, pressure on the ribs, or lifting the arm away from the rib cage.

Chiropractic manipulation is the treatment of choice in most cases. Rib subluxations usually resolve in 1-3 treatments. Sometimes, soft tissue massage, proprioceptive taping, topical analgesics, or the use of ice or heat may enhance healing.

Thoracic Disc Herniation

Herniated discs in the mid-back are very uncommon, accounting for only about 1-2% of all spinal disc problems seen, and have been estimated to effect 1 in every million patients.

People with this disorder can suffer from pain in the mid-back only, or may have numbness or pain in the chest or side. As such, these can often be confused with disorders in the heart, lungs, or abdomen. For this reason, a thorough workup from your doctor to rule out serious pathologies is crucial before confirming that a thoracic disc problem is responsible for causing pain.

Non-surgical treatment, such as chiropractic care, is usually the most appropriate for thoracic disc disorders. A 1993 article on thoracic disc herniations in *Neurosurgical Clinics of North America*, stated that "a conservative therapeutic plan is recommended." Exercise, medication, manipulation, traction, nutritional support, and physiotherapy are often used to decrease pain associated with thoracic disc disorders. Surgery for thoracic disc problems is extremely rare, although various forms of injections (epidurals, nerve blocks, etc.) may offer relief in more severe cases.

A Word About Stress

When most people become stressed, they unconsciously contract their muscles, in particular, the muscles in their back. This 'muscle guarding' is a survival response designed to protect against injury. In today's world where we are not exposed to physical danger most of the time, muscle guarding still occurs whenever we become emotionally stressed. The areas most affected are the muscles of the neck, upper back, and low back. For most of us, the particular muscle affected by stress is the trapezius muscle, where daily stress usually leads to chronic tightness and the development of trigger points.

The two most effective ways to reduce the physical effects of stress is to increase your activity level (exercise) and by deep breathing exercises. When you decrease the physical effects of stress, you can substantially reduce the amount of tightness and pain in your upper back and neck.

Treating Neck and Upper Back Pain with Chiropractic

In order to achieve the goal of reducing or eliminating upper back and neck pain, it is necessary to re-establish normal posture, mobility, strength, and coordination of the spinal vertebrae, joints, and muscles. Numerous studies conducted by universities and funded by the U.S. government have shown repeatedly that chiropractic adjustments are one of the most effective means of treating problems in the spine, especially in the low back and neck regions.

Exercises for Your Neck and Upper Back

Because you have to support the weight of your head on top of your highly unstable neck, it is critical that your neck and upper back muscles be flexible and strong. It is important, however, that when you start exercising a particular muscle or muscle group, that it is free from spasm and trigger points in order to avoid irritating the muscle tissue. There are a number of exercises and stretches for your neck and upper back listed later on in this book. If you have not done these exercises before, be sure to start off slow and light, and build up the intensity over several weeks. This will help you to avoid injuries to your muscles while improving your health.

4

Headaches

"A quiet mind cureth all."

- Robert Burton

Headaches affect just about everyone at some point, and they can present themselves in many different ways. Some people only experience pain in one part of their head or behind their eyes; some people experience a pounding sensation inside their whole head. Some people experience nausea while others do not. The pain itself may be dull or sharp and may last for anywhere from a few minutes to a few days. Fortunately, very few headaches have serious underlying causes, but those that do require urgent medical attention.

Headaches are common, but they are not normal. Although the International Headache Society has classified 129 different types of headaches, the most common headaches come from the muscles (muscle tension), blood vessels (migraines), spinal joints (cervicogenic), or systemic conditions, such as high blood pressure and diabetes.

Muscular Tension Headaches

Tension headaches are the most common type of headache, affecting upwards of 75% of all headache sufferers. Most people describe a tension headache as a constant dull, achy feeling either on one or both sides of the head. A tension headache is often described as a feeling of a tight band or dull ache around the head or behind the eyes. These headaches usually begin slowly and gradually, often in the middle or toward the end of the day.

Tension headaches, or stress headaches, can last from 30 minutes to several days. In some cases, chronic tension headaches may persist for many months. Although the pain can at times be severe, tension headaches are usually not associated with other symptoms such as throbbing, nausea, or vomiting.

The most common cause of tension headaches is subluxations in the upper back and neck, especially the upper neck, usually in combination with active trigger points. When the top cervical vertebrae lose their normal motion or position, a small muscle called the rectus capitis posterior minor (RCPM) muscle goes into spasm. This small muscle has a tendon which slips between the upper neck and the base of the skull and attaches to a thin tissue called the dura mater that covers the brain. Although the brain itself has no feeling, the dura mater is very pain-sensitive. Consequently, when the RCPM muscle goes into spasm and its tendon tugs at the dura mater, a headache occurs.

Another cause of tension type headaches comes from referred pain from trigger points in the sternocleidomastoid (SCM) or levator muscle on the side of the neck. These are much more common in people who have muscle damage in the neck caused by a whiplash injury.

Migraine Headaches

Each year, about 25 million people in the U.S. experience migraine headaches. About 75% of migraine sufferers are women. Migraines are intense, throbbing headaches that are often associated with nausea and sensitivity to light or noise. They can last from as little as a few hours to as long as a few days. Many of those who suffer from migraines experience visual symptoms called an "aura" just prior to an attack that is sometimes described as seeing flashing lights. Sometimes, it appears as though everything has taken on a dream-like appearance.

Migraine headaches tend to run in families and most sufferers have their first attack before age 30, supporting the notion that there is a genetic component to them. Some people

The Three Major Types of Headaches

	Cervicogenic & Tension	Migraine	Cluster
Gradual Onset	X		
Rapid Onset		X	X
Throbbing Pain		X	X
Dull, Aching Pain	X		
Stress Can Elicit Headache	X	X	X
Diet Can Elicit Headache		X	X
Affects Mostly Women		X	
Affects Mostly Men			X
Short Duration			X
Long Duration	X	X	
Occur Frequently	X		
Often Disabling		X	X
Often Associated With Nausea		X	
Muscular Involvement	X		
Vascular Involvement		X	X
Spinal Involvement	X		

have attacks several times a month; others have less than one a year. Many people find that migraine attacks occur less frequently and become less severe as they get older.

Migraine headaches are caused by a constriction of the blood vessels in the brain, followed by a reflexive over-dilation. During the constriction of the blood vessels, there is a decrease in blood flow, which is what leads to the visual symptoms that many people experience. Even in people who don't experience the classic migraine aura, there is a sense that an attack is imminent. Once the blood vessels dilate, there is a rapid increase in blood pressure inside the head. It is this increased pressure that leads to the pounding headache. Each time the heart beats, it sends another shock wave through the carotid arteries in the neck up into the brain.

There are many theories about why the blood vessels constrict in the first place, but no one knows for sure. What we do know is that there are a number of things that can trigger migraines such as lack of sleep, stress, flickering lights, strong odors, changing weather patterns, and several foods - especially foods that are high in an amino acid called 'tyramine.' At the end of this chapter, I have listed a number of foods that are most likely to trigger migraines as well as some lifestyle changes that you can make to reduce the likelihood that you will trigger a migraine headache.

Cervicogenic Headaches

Headaches originating in the neck have been shown to be responsible for almost 20% of the headaches in patients who have more than five headaches per month. This type of headache impairs function and reduces quality of life as much, or more, than migraine headaches.

Patients with cervicogenic headaches are likely to have neck pain or tenderness in addition to the headache itself. These people often describe their pain as "piercing" or "dull."

Their symptoms begin in the middle of upper neck and can radiate into the sides of the head near the temples or behind the eyes. These headaches often become more severe once they radiate from the neck into the head and can last from hours to weeks. People with these headaches are likely to have impaired motion of the neck, often finding it difficult to bend, the neck forward or rotate the head from side to side.

Cluster Headaches

Cluster headaches are typically very short-duration, excruciating headaches and are usually felt on one side of the head behind the eyes. Cluster headaches affect about one million people in the United States and, unlike migraines, are much more common in men. This is the only type of headache that tends to occur at night. The reason that they are called 'cluster' headaches is that they tend to occur one to four times per day over a period of several days. After one cluster of headaches is over, it may be months or even years before they occur again. Like migraines, cluster headaches are likely to be related to an over-dilation of the blood vessels in the brain, causing a localized increase in pressure.

Chiropractic Care for Headaches

Chiropractic treatment of headaches is very patient-specific but generally involves a two-step approach of nonpharmacologic treatments such as manipulation, soft tissue treatments, biofeedback, exercise and nutritional advice, along with avoiding triggers that cause headaches in the first place.

Numerous research studies have shown that chiropractic adjustments are very effective for treating tension headaches, especially headaches that originate in the neck.

A report released in 2001 by researchers at the Duke University Evidence-Based Practice Center in Durham, North Carolina, found that "spinal manipulation resulted in almost immediate improvement for those headaches that originate in the neck, and had significantly fewer side effects and longer-lasting relief of tension-type headache than commonly prescribed medications."

These findings support an earlier study published in *The Journal of Manipulative and Physiological Therapeutics*, which found spinal manipulative therapy to be very effective for treating tension headaches. This study also found that even those patients who stopped chiropractic treatment after only four weeks continued to experience a sustained benefit in contrast to those patients who received pain medication.

In 2003, a double-blind, placebo-controlled study compared migraine patients undergoing chiropractic manipulation versus electric muscle stimulation. After only two months of treatment, the severity and frequency of migraine headaches was significantly less in the chiropractic patients. The patients receiving chiropractic care continued to have a measurable improvement in symptoms compared to the control group two months after the treatments.

The Journal of the Neuromusculoskeletal System reported in 2002 that within nine chiropractic treatments, sufferers of tension-type headaches averaged 64% improvement in their symptoms.

Spinal manipulation involves a hands-on approach to restoring mobility to spinal joints in the neck and upper back and often helps to reduce nerve irritation and restore normal curvature in the neck, relieve muscle spasm, and improve circulation.

Several soft tissue techniques such as NIMMO trigger point therapy, proprioceptive neuromuscular facilitation, and Strain-Counterstrain Technique are also useful. These low-force therapies are used to release muscle spasms in the upper back, neck, and in the suboccipital area at the base of the skull. The suboccipital area, in particular, has been implicated in most tension or cervicogenic headaches, which is why many patients report feeling their headache begins in their neck or back of the head.

Each individual's case is different and requires a thorough evaluation before a proper course of chiropractic care can be determined. However, in most cases of tension headaches, significant improvement is accomplished through manipulation of the upper two cervical vertebrae, coupled with adjustments to the junction between the cervical and thoracic spine. This is also helpful in most cases of migraine headaches as long as food and lifestyle triggers are avoided as well.

Avoid Headache Triggers

• Stress may be a trigger, but certain foods, odors, menstrual periods, and changes in weather are among many factors that may also trigger headaches.

• Emotional factors such as depression, anxiety, frustration, letdown, and even nervous excitement may be associated with developing headaches.

• Keeping a headache diary will help you determine whether factors such as food or changes in weather and/or mood have any relationship to your headache pattern.

• Repeated exposure to nitrite compounds can result in a dull, pounding headache that may be accompanied by a flushed face. Nitrites, which dilate blood vessels, are found in such products as hot dogs, sausage, brats, bologna, and other processed meats.

• Eating foods prepared with monosodium glutamate (MSG) can result in headaches. Soy sauce, meat tenderizer, and a variety of packaged foods contain this chemical, which is touted as a flavor enhancer.

• Headaches can also result from exposure to poisons such as insecticides and herbicides. Children who ingest flakes of lead paint may develop headaches.

- Foods that are high in the amino acid tyramine should also be avoided, such as ripened cheeses (such as cheddar or brie), chocolate, as well as any pickled or fermented foods.

5

Whiplash

"Health is the greatest gift, contentment the greatest wealth, and faithfulness the best relationship."
-Buddha

The term *whiplash* was first used in 1928 to define an injury mechanism of sudden hyperextension followed by an immediate hyperflexion of the neck, which results in damage to the muscles, ligaments, and tendons – especially those that support the head. Today, we know that whiplash injuries frequently do not result from hyperextension or hyperflexion (extension and flexion beyond normal physiological limits) but rather an extremely rapid extension and flexion.

Due to their complicated nature and profound impact on people's lives, few topics in health care generate as much controversy as whiplash injuries. Unlike a broken bone where a simple x-ray can validate the presence of the fracture and standards of care can direct a health care professional to the best way in which to handle the injury, whiplash injuries involve an unpredictable combination of nervous system, muscles, joints, and connective tissue disruption that is not simple to diagnose and can be even more of a challenge to treat. In order to help you understand the nature of whiplash injuries and how they should be treated, it is necessary to spend a bit of time discussing the mechanics of how whiplash injuries occur.

The Four Phases of a Whiplash Injury

During a rear-end automobile collision, your body goes through an extremely rapid and intense acceleration and deceleration. In fact, all four phases of a whiplash injury occur in less than one-half of a second! At each phase, there is a different force acting on the body that contributes to the overall injury, and with such a sudden and forceful movement, damage to the vertebrae, nerves, discs, muscles, and ligaments of your neck and spine can be substantial.

Phase One Whiplash

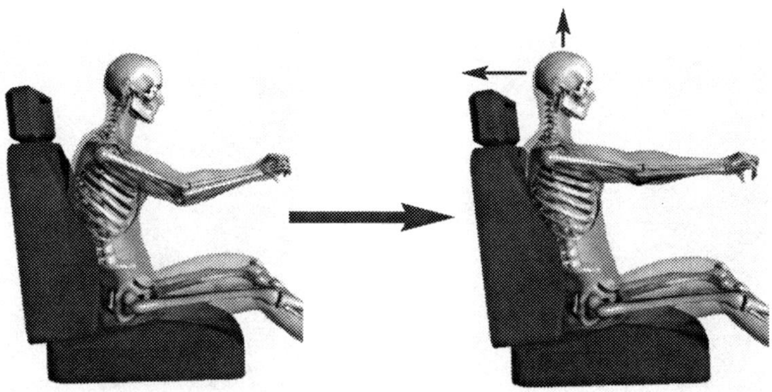

During this phase, your car begins to be pushed out from under you and your mid-back and neck begin to straighten. This causes upward compressive and shearing forces in the neck.

Phase One

During this first phase, your car begins to be pushed out from under you, causing your mid-back to be flattened against the back of your seat. This results in an upward force in your cervical spine, compressing your discs and joints. As your seat back begins to accelerate your torso forward, your head also moves backward, creating a shearing force in your neck. If your head restraint is properly adjusted, the distance your head travels backward is limited. However, most of the damage to the spine will occur before your head reaches your head restraint. Studies have shown that head restraints only reduce the risk of injury by 11-20%.

Phase Two Whiplash

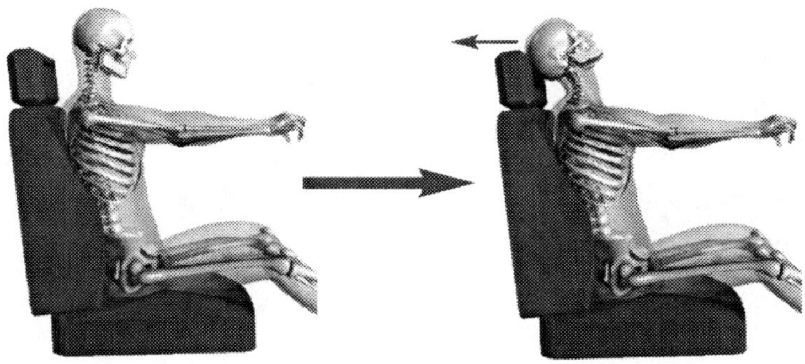

During this phase, your head continues to move backward into extension, creating a powerful shearing force in the neck. This shearing, combined with the compression of the spine in the neck, causes substantial injury.

Phase Two

During phase two, your torso has reached peak acceleration - 1.5 to 2 times that of your vehicle itself - but your head has not yet begun to accelerate forward, and in fact continues to move rearward. An abnormal S-curve develops in your cervical spine as your seat back recoils forward, much like a springboard, adding to the forward acceleration of the torso. Unfortunately, this forward seat back recoil occurs while your head is still moving backward, resulting in a shearing force in the neck that is one of the more damaging aspects of a whiplash injury. Many of the bone, joint, nerve, disc, and TMJ injuries that we see clinically occur during this phase.

Phase Three Whiplash

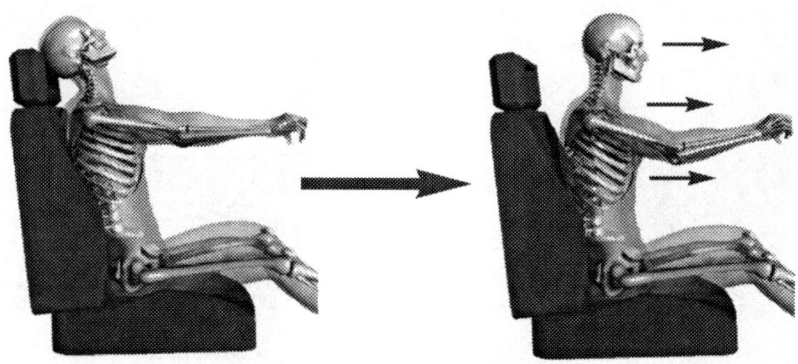

During this phase, your head and torso are projected forward from the recoil of your seat as the seat is projected forward. As you are wearing a seat belt, any slack in the belt is taken up.

Phase Three

During the third phase, your torso is now descending back down in your seat and your head and neck are at their peak forward acceleration. At the same time, your car is slowing down. If you released the pressure on your brake pedal during the first phases of the collision, it will likely be reapplied during this phase. Reapplication of the brake causes your car to slow down even quicker and increases the severity of the flexion injury of your neck. As you move forward in your seat, any slack in your seat belt and shoulder harness is taken up.

Phase Four Whiplash

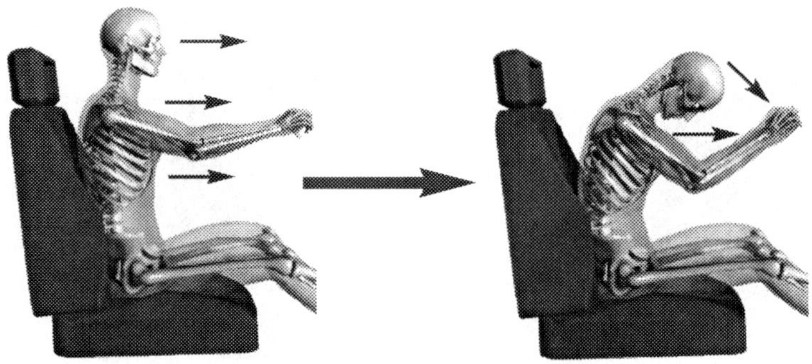

During this phase, your head and torso continue to be projected forward, but your torso is kept from moving forward by your seat belt. The forward energy is then transferred through your neck causing it to go into hyperflextion.

Phase Four

This is probably the most damaging phase of the whiplash phenomenon. In this fourth phase, your torso is stopped by your seat belt and shoulder restraint and your head is free to move forward unimpeded. This results in a violent forward-bending motion of your neck, straining the muscles and ligaments, tearing fibers in the spinal discs, and forcing vertebrae out of their normal position. Your spinal cord and nerve roots get stretched and irritated, and your brain can strike the inside of your skull. This can cause a mild to moderate brain injury. If you are not properly restrained by your seat

Resolution

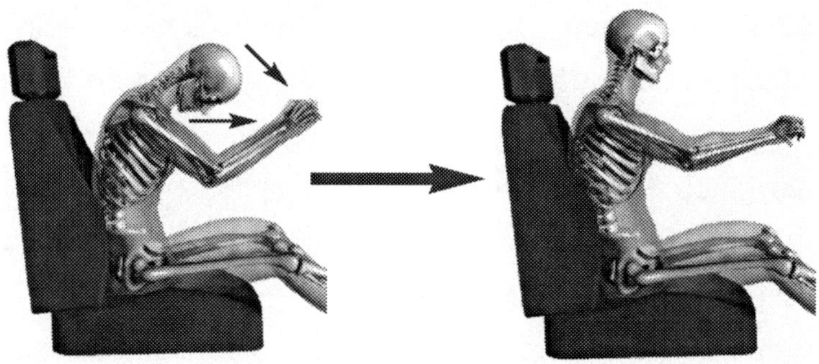

The resolution phase is when the energy from the collision has dissipated and your body returns to a neutral position from the hyperflexion of phase four.

harness, you may suffer a concussion, or more severe brain injury, from striking the steering wheel or windshield.

Resolution

Once the collision forces dissipate, your body goes back into a neutral position. The entire whiplash injury process from initial contact to the resolution phase takes place in less than one-half second. If a secondary collision occurs, the body goes through this process again, further injuring damaged tissues.

Injuries Resulting from Whiplash Trauma

Whiplash injuries can manifest in a wide variety of ways, including neck pain, headaches, fatigue, upper back and shoulder pain, cognitive changes, and low back pain. Due to the fact that numerous factors play into the overall whiplash trauma, such as direction of impact, speed of the vehicles involved, as well as sex, age, and physical condition, it is impossible to predict the pattern of symptoms that each individual will suffer. Additionally, whiplash symptoms commonly have a delayed onset, often taking weeks or months to present. There are, however, a number of conditions that are very common among those who have suffered from whiplash trauma.

Neck Pain

Neck pain is the single most common complaint in whiplash trauma, being reported by over 90% of patients. Often this pain radiates across the shoulders, up into the head, and down between the shoulder blades. Whiplash injuries tend to affect all of the tissues in the neck, including the facet joints and discs between the vertebrae, as well as all of the muscles, ligaments, and nerves.

Facet joint pain is the most common cause of neck pain following a car accident. Facet joint pain is usually felt on the back of the neck, just to the right or left of center, and is often tender to the touch. Facet joint pain cannot be visualized on x-rays or MRIs. It can only be diagnosed by physical palpation of the area, or with injections to numb the joint.

Disc injury is also a common cause of neck pain, especially chronic pain. The outer wall of the disc (called the annulus) is made up of bundles of fibers that can be torn during a whiplash trauma. These tears can lead to disc degeneration or herniation, resulting in irritation or compression of the nerves running through the area. This compression or irritation commonly leads to radiating pain into the arms, shoulders, and upper back, and may result in muscle weakness.

Damage to the muscles and ligaments in the neck and upper back are the major cause of the pain experienced in the first few weeks following a whiplash injury, and is the main reason why you experience stiffness and restricted range of motion. As the muscles have a chance to heal, they typically don't cause as much pain as they contribute to abnormal movement. Damage to the ligaments often results in abnormal movement and instability.

Headaches

After neck pain, headaches are the most prevalent complaint among those suffering from whiplash injury, affecting more than 50% of all people. While some headaches are actually the result of direct brain injury, most are related to injury of the muscles, ligaments, and facet joints of the cervical spine, which refer pain to the head. Because of this, it is important to treat the supporting structures of your neck in order to help alleviate your headaches.

Temporomandibular Joint Dysfunction

A less common, but very debilitating disorder that results from whiplash is temporomandibular joint dysfunction (TMD). TMD usually begins as pain, clicking and popping noises in the jaw during movement. If not properly evaluated and treated, TMD problems can continue to worsen and lead to headaches, facial pain, ear pain, and difficulty chewing. Chiropractors have been trained to treat TMD problems and often begin treatment for this on a patient's first visit.

Brain Injury

Mild to moderate brain injury is common following a whiplash injury due to the forces on the brain during the four phases mentioned earlier. The human brain is a very soft structure, suspended in a watery fluid called cerebrospinal fluid. When the brain is forced forward and backward in the skull, the brain bounces off the inside of the skull, leading to bruising or bleeding in the brain itself. In some cases, patients temporarily lose consciousness and have symptoms of a mild concussion. More often, there is no loss of consciousness, but

How Brain Injuries Occur

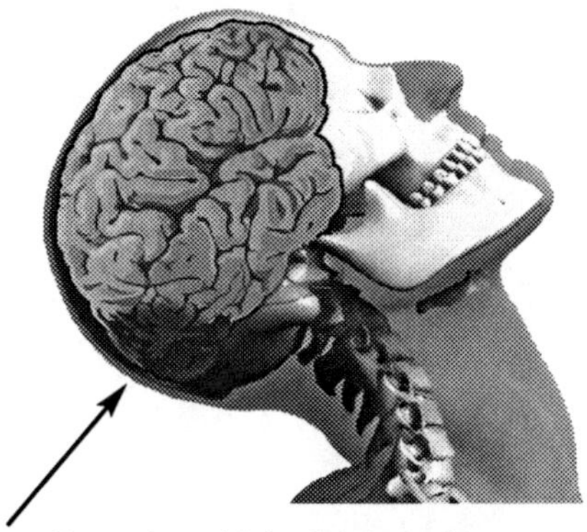

During Phase Two of a whiplash injury, the posterior portion of the brain strikes the rear portion of the inside of the skull.

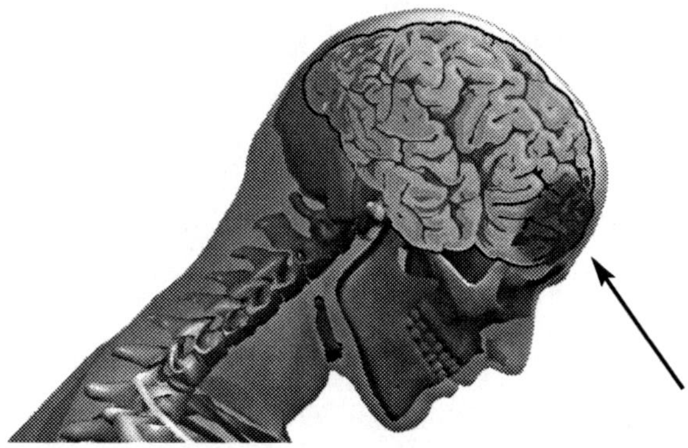

During Phase Four of a whiplash injury, the anterior portion of the brain strikes the front portion of the inside of the skull.

This type of brain injury is technically known as a "coup counter-coup" injury - the "coup" being the initial striking of the posterior of the brain, followed by a rebounding "counter-coup" injury when the anterior portion of the brain strikes the front of the skull - and commonly leads to measurable cognitive changes, sometimes permanently.

patients complain of mild confusion or disorientation just after the crash. The long-term consequences of a mild brain injury can include mild confusion, difficulty concentrating, sleep disturbances, irritability, forgetfulness, loss of sex drive, depression, and emotional instability. Although less common, the nerves responsible for your sense of smell, taste, and even your vision may be affected.

Dizziness

Dizziness following a whiplash injury usually results from injury to the facet joints of the cervical spine, although in some cases injury to the brain or brain stem may be a factor as well. Typically, this dizziness is very temporary and improves significantly over time with treatment.

Low Back Pain

Although most people consider whiplash to be an injury of the neck, the low back is also commonly injured. In fact, low back pain is found in more than half of rear impact-collisions in which injury was reported, and almost three-quarters of all side-impact crashes. This is mostly due to the fact that the low back experiences a tremendous compression during the first two phases of a whiplash injury, even though it does not have the degree of flexion-extension injury experienced in the neck.

Recovery from Whiplash

With proper care, many mild whiplash injuries heal within four to nine months. However, more than 20% of those who suffer from whiplash injuries continue to suffer from pain, weakness, or restricted movement two years after their accident. Unfortunately, many of these people will continue to suffer from some level of disability or pain for many years after that, if not for the rest of their lives.

Just as there are many different things that influence how severe a whiplash injury will be, there are numerous factors that have an impact on how completely an individual will recover, including the following:

- symptoms persisting beyond six months
- severity of ligament, disc, nerve, or joint injury
- delay in initiating treatment
- recurrent flare-ups of pain
- age over 65
- sex: females are at a higher risk of injury
- head restraint more than 2" away from the head
- whether the occupant was in a small car
- alcohol intoxication at time of automobile accident
- prior whiplash injury or degenerative changes
- experiencing numbness or tingling after the accident
- a cervical collar used for more than two weeks

Any of these conditions will increase the likelihood of a longer recovery period and increase the risk of permanent injury. Although some of these factors are beyond your control, such as your age, most of them are under your control, especially alcohol consumption, the position of your head restraint, and delaying initial chiropractic treatment. After many years of treating people with chronic whiplash injury pain, we know how disabling it can be. The sooner you begin treatment, the better your chances are for a full recovery.

6

Diagnosis and Treatment

"You can set yourself up to be sick, or you can choose to stay well."

-Dr. Wayne Dyer

Getting to the bottom of what is causing your neck or back pain involves three steps: 1) a health history; 2) a physical exam; and 3) diagnostic imaging, such as x-rays or magnetic resonance imaging (MRI).

A thorough medical history and physical exam can usually identify any dangerous conditions that may be associated with your back pain. You will be asked to describe the nature, location, severity, as well as the onset of your pain, the duration of your symptoms, and any health conditions that might be

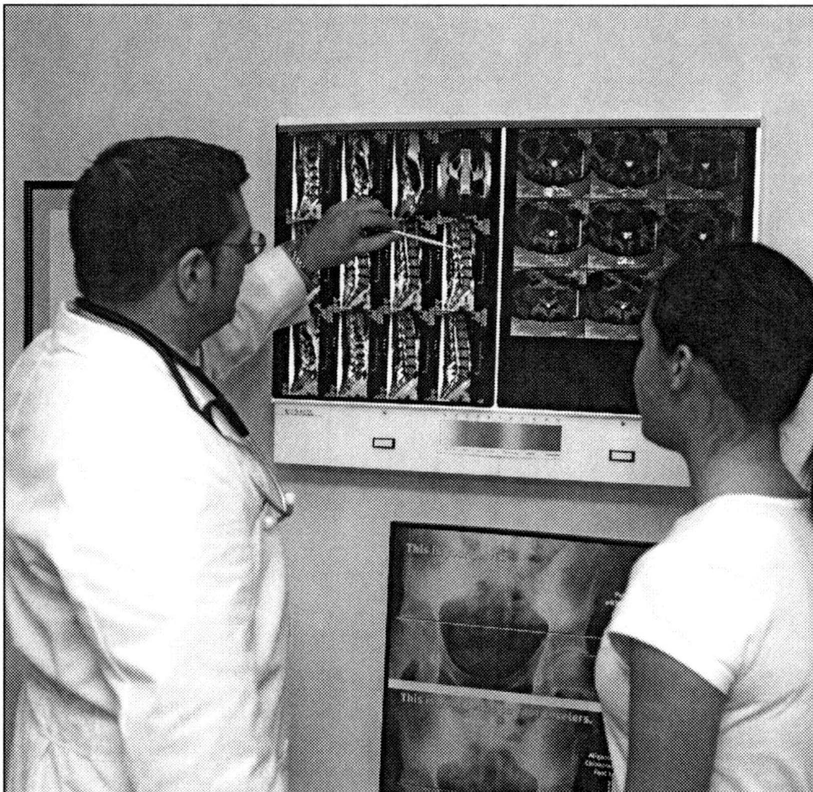

Understanding why you have pain, and what can be done for it, is a function of communication between doctor and patient.

related to the pain. Depending on what is found during the history and exam, imaging tests may be necessary to diagnose the source of your pain and to rule out more serious conditions.

Your Medical History

During the medical history, you will be asked questions about the nature of your pain and about any health problems you and close family members have had. Questions may include

- Have you had back pain before? If so, what was the cause?
- Are there any activities or positions that ease or aggravate your pain?
- Have you recently fallen or injured your back?
- Does your back feel better – or hurt worse – when you lie down?
- Is your pain worse or better at a certain time of day?
- Do you or any family members have any diseases that affect the spine?
- Do you have pain, numbness, or tingling in either or both of your arms or legs?
- What treatments have you had for your current problem?

The information found in the history is usually enough to give your chiropractor a good indication as to the cause of your back pain. At the very least, it will help your doctor determine which diagnostic tests need to be performed. The more specific information that you can provide, the more accurately a diagnosis can be reached after the exam and diagnostic imaging.

Your Physical Exam

A thorough physical exam is critical to confirm, or change, the diagnosis of what may be causing your low back pain. During an exam for low back pain, your doctor may

- Watch you stand and walk.
- Check your reflexes.
- Check for muscle strength and sensation.
- Check for signs of nerve root irritation.
- Check your range of motion in your spine, arms, and legs.
- Check areas of tenderness, heat, or spasm.

Often, the cause of your pain can be determined with a physical and medical history alone. However, depending on what the history and exam show, your doctor may order additional diagnostic imaging, such as an x-ray. A variety of diagnostic imaging methods are available to confirm the cause of your pain.

X-ray

An x-ray is often the first imaging technique used, looking for fractured or dislocated bones or an injured vertebra, as well as any instability or abnormal posture. X-rays are not routinely necessary for most episodes of acute back pain. They are mainly used to detect serious underlying structural, pathologic conditions.

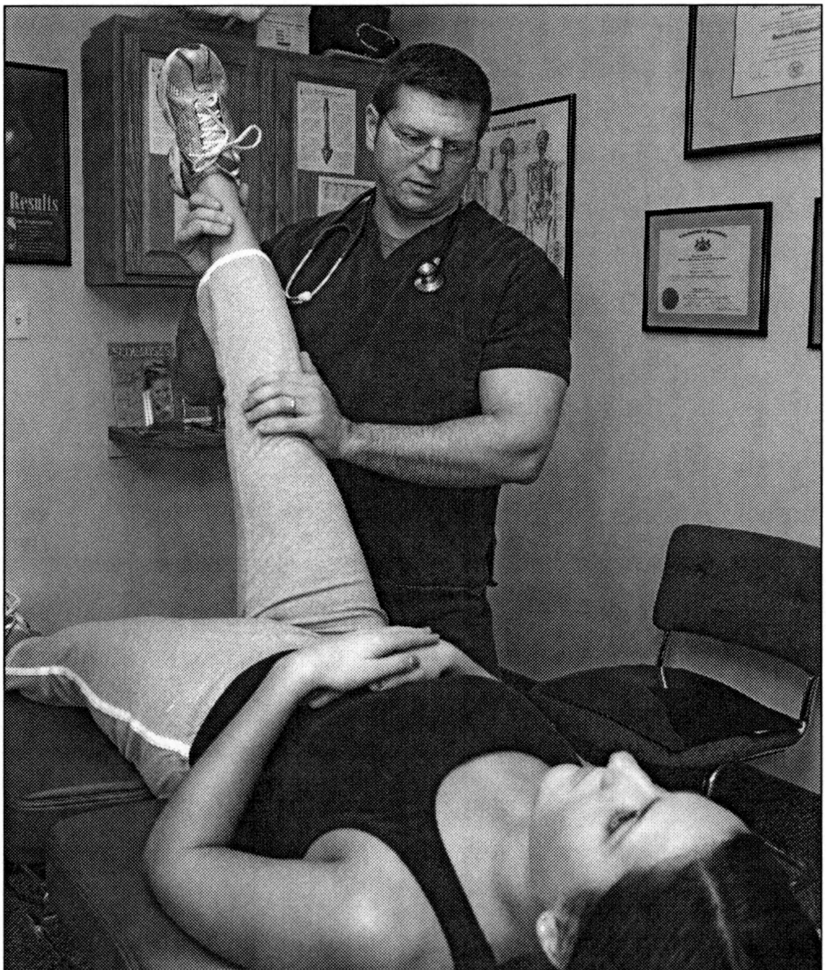

A thorough exam is an integral part of establishing an accurate diagnosis.

There are clinical guidelines that dictate when x-rays are necessary, such as in cases of suspected fracture, history of cancer or surgery, physical deformities, and trauma. Sometimes x-rays are ordered after an adequate trial of treatment has failed to provide any relief.

During an x-ray, a technician passes a highly focused beam of low-dose ionized radiation through the back and takes pictures that, within minutes, show the bony structures of the body. Injured muscles and ligaments or painful conditions such as a bulging disc are not visible on conventional x-rays.

Computed Tomography (CT)

Like an x-ray, a computed tomography (CT) scan works by shooting an x-ray beam through the body. Instead of the x-rays exposing a sheet of film, a computer is used to collect and reformat the image into cross sections of the spine. During a CT, x-rays are passed through the body at various angles and are detected by a computerized scanner to produce two-dimensional images of the internal structures of the back.

CT imaging of the lumbar spine provides superior anatomic imaging of the bony structures of the spine and are also useful to assess the soft tissues of the spine such as discs, ligaments, nerve roots and fat. They are usually used when a fracture, disc rupture, spinal stenosis, or damage to vertebrae are suspected as a cause of low back pain. This diagnostic exam is generally conducted at an imaging center or hospital.

Magnetic Resonance Imaging(MRI)

A magnetic resonance imaging (MRI) scan is a completely different technology from an x-ray or a CT scan. Instead of passing x-rays through the body, an MRI scanner places your body into a magnetic field to temporarily realign the water molecules in your body's tissues. Radio waves are then passed through the body to trigger a resonance signal at different angles within the body. A computer processes this resonance into either a three-dimensional picture or a two-dimensional "slice" of the tissue being scanned. MRI scans are much better at differentiating between bone, soft tissues, and fluid-filled spaces than either x-rays or CT scan.

An MRI scan is particularly useful as an aid in the assessment of certain back conditions by providing detail of the spinal disc (such as degenerative disc disease, spondylolisthesis) and nerve roots (such as lumbar disc herniation, lumbar spinal stenosis). MRI scans are also useful to rule out tumors or spinal infections. As with other tests, the use of an MRI is reserved for those patients not responding as expected to treatment.

Discography

A discography, or discogram, is an enhanced x-ray examination of the pads of cartilage (intervertebral discs) that separate the bones in your spine (vertebrae). During this procedure, dye is injected into the center of one or more discs, which makes the discs more visible on x-ray film. A discogram is used to detect structural damage in a disc and to help determine whether a disc is causing pain. The test can show if a disc has begun to rupture or has tears in its outer shell. By injecting fluid into the disc, the doctor can determine if the disc is painful.

A discogram involves the injection of a special contrast dye into a spinal disc thought to be causing low back pain. The dye outlines the damaged areas on x-rays taken following the injection. This procedure is often suggested for patients who are considering lumbar surgery or whose pain has not responded to conventional treatments. It can be useful for patients who have not responded to a well-coordinated chiropractic rehabilitation program or who have normal or equivocal MRI findings.

Electrodiagnostics: Electromyography (EMG) and Somatosensory Evoked Potential (SSEP)

Electrodiagnostic studies, including electromyography (EMG) and somatosensory evoked potential studies (SSEPs), are an extension of the history and physical examination. These studies are helpful in the evaluation of patients with limb pain where the diagnosis remains unclear (e.g. peripheral neuropathy versus a radiculopathy). They are also helpful in excluding other causes of sensory and motor disturbances, such as peripheral neuropathy and motor neuron disease.

EMG assesses the electrical activity in a nerve and can detect if muscle weakness results from an injury or other problems with the nerves that control the muscles. During an

EMG, very fine needles are inserted in the effected muscles to measure electrical activity transmitted from the brain or spinal cord to a particular area of the body. With nerve conduction studies, there are two sets of electrodes that are placed on the skin over the muscles. The first set gives the patient a mild shock to stimulate the nerve that runs to a particular muscle. The second set of electrodes is used to make a recording of the nerve's electrical signals, and from this information the doctor can determine if there is nerve damage.

Somatosensory evoked potential studies (SSEPs) also involve two sets of electrodes — one set to stimulate a sensory nerve and the other set on the scalp to record the speed of nerve signal transmissions to the brain. SSEPs are used to assess nerve conduction across the spinal cord. If the spinal cord is significantly pinched, the electrical signals will travel slower than usual. They may also be used to monitor spinal cord function during surgical procedures, although since the spinal cord ends before the lumbar spine, this is usually of limited value during lumbar spinal surgery and it is used more often in cervical (neck) or thoracic (chest) spine surgery.

Bone Scans

Bone scans are used to diagnose and monitor infection, fracture, or metabolic disorders in bone. During a bone scan, a small amount of radioactive material is injected into the bloodstream. This radioactive material tends to accumulate in areas of bone where there is a lot of metabolic action, such as an area where there is a fracture, tumor, or other problem. A bone scan is sometimes performed to rule out an inflammatory process (such as a tumor or infection) or an occult fracture (small fracture not seen on an x-ray).

Scanner-generated images are then sent to a computer to be analyzed and displayed. A positive bone scan, indicating some abnormal metabolic process, is typically confirmed by additional imaging such as MRI or CT, which provide for greater detail of the spine.

In addition, other tests, such as doppler ultrasound to rule out blood clots in the leg that can mimic sciatica, bone density scans to rule out osteoporosis, bone scans to assess for a fracture or tumors, or blood work to rule out systemic diseases, are commonly used by Doctors of Chiropractic.

As stated earlier, a thorough physical examination is usually adequate to provide your doctor with a diagnosis. Most back pain is mechanical, meaning its cause can be found through orthopedic tests, ranges of motion, and the other components of a thorough physical examination.

When in doubt or unsure, modern medicine has afforded us the ability to use the tests explained above. A responsible chiropractic clinician is trained to utilize these tests when they are appropriate, and when they offer your doctor information that will steer the course of treatment in the right direction.

7

Chiropractic Care

"The high usage of painkillers reflects a failure of modern medicine to convince people that they can overcome benign pain with normal activity, guided exercise, and other nonpharmacological measures."

-Vert Mooney, M.D.

What is Chiropractic?

Chiropractic is a branch of the healing arts that focuses on the relationship between structure and function in the human body. The term *chiropractic* comes from the Greek words *cheiro* and *praktikos*, meaning "done by hand." The purpose of chiropractic treatment is to uncover the cause of your symptoms, not to merely cover up these symptoms.

Doctors of Chiropractic do not prescribe medications or perform surgery. Rather, they draw from a wealth of training and resources to treat patients through conservative (non-invasive) treatments. Chiropractic care is aimed at restoring and maintaining normal structure and function of the joints, muscles, and nervous system.

Chiropractic in the 21st Century

Once thought of as "alternative" or "complementary" to traditional medical care, chiropractic treatment has, over the past decade, become part of mainstream health care. Over 15 million people utilize chiropractic care, and chiropractors are seen in private practice, within hospitals, and in multidisciplinary clinics throughout the world.

Doctors of Chiropractic serve on insurance boards, teach in prominent medical schools, and testify as experts in forensic cases. Chiropractic has become integrated into the modern healthcare system and is, in fact, more recognized and accepted than many other nontraditional therapies. Chiropractors are an integral part of a health care team in the 21st century and are an invaluable resource in the non-operative treatment of pain.

Common Forms of Treatment Used by Doctors of Chiropractic

Chiropractors use a variety of techniques and procedures in the treatment of spinal problems and for the promotion of overall health and wellness. The most commonly used methods of treatment in my office are discussed in this chapter. As with any healing art, the type of treatment is based on a variety of factors that are assessed when a history is taken and the patient is examined.

Chiropractic Manipulative Therapy (CMT)

Perhaps the most common treatment associated with chiropractic is the use of spinal manipulation. This procedure is sometimes referred to as Chiropractic Manipulative Therapy (CMT) or "adjustments" because the spine is being "adjusted" to create movement and restore its range of motion. The objective of a chiropractic adjustment is to reduce subluxation, which results in increased range of motion, reduced nerve irritability, and improved function.

During an adjustment, a trained Doctor of Chiropractic manually administers a small thrust to a spinal joint. This may be associated with a cracking or popping sound, which has been shown in research studies to be a release of small pockets of air bubbles (oxygen, nitrogen, and carbon dioxide) within the spinal joint. The sound is simply a release of gas, similar to opening a can of soda. The sensation with a chiropractic adjustment is usually one of relief.

Contrary to popular belief, chiropractic manipulation is not an attempt to fix a "bone out of place." In the early days of chiropractic, the "bone out of place" model was used to explain the concept of the Vertebral Subluxation Complex (VSC) and should not be taken literally. The VSC has been discussed in detail in Chapter 3. It is important to remember that spinal joints that are functioning properly are not painful and are less likely to become injured or degenerate.

Scientific evidence of the effectiveness of chiropractic manipulation has been demonstrated over and over. It has been proven to be effective in treating mechanical disturbances in the spine, and may have wider positive effects on health and wellness.

Again, we look to sound research studies to illustrate what chiropractic manipulation has been shown to do.

• Increase the size of the spinal canal. This provides more room for the spinal cord, and decreases the effects of spinal conditions that narrow this important space (such as spinal stenosis, degenerative disc disease, and facet syndrome). (*Journal of the Neuromusculoskeletal System*, 1998)

• Gap open the spinal facet joints (A common source of pain in the back and neck) as seen on MRI and studies at the National University of Health Sciences. (*Spine*, 2002; 2459-2466)

• Increase range of motion in the spine. Spinal joint range of motion increases with chiropractic treatment. This is especially important in cases of injury, trauma, or degenerative changes, which often cause loss of motion in the spine. (*Journal of Manipulative & Physiological Therapeutics,* 1992;15:495-500)

• Reduce spinal pain. Chiropractic treatments have been shown to effect the levels of pain. (*American Journal of Physical Medicine*, 1984;63:217-25)

• Increase pain tolerance in spinal muscles. These muscles, which are often effected with injury, degenerative disorders, disc problems, or VSC, actually become more resistant to pain after chiropractic treatments. (*Journal of Manipulative & Physiological Therapeutics*, 1990;13:13-16)

• Reduce the electrical activity and tension in muscles. The excitability of back muscles is decreased after a chiropractic treatment. This relaxation often eases pain and increases function. (*Journal of Manipulative & Physiological Therapeutics,* 1987;10:300-04)

• Reduce blood pressure. Chiropractic treatments have been shown to positively effect blood pressure. (*Journal of Manipulative & Physiological Therapeutics*, 1988;11:484-488)

• Increase plasma endorphins and melatonin levels. Melatonin has been used to treat insomnia as well as boosting the immune system. Endorphins are naturally occurring neurotransmitters that are analgesic, meaning they help alleviate pain. The levels of these chemicals actually increases after a chiropractic treatment. (*Journal of Manipulative & Physiological Therapeutics*, 1992;15:83-89 & 1986;9:119-123)

• Decrease the excitability and irritation of spinal nerves. Chiropractic treatment has been shown to reduce the hyper-excited and irritable states of nerves. (*Spine,* 2000;25:2519-25)

• Down-regulate (decrease) inflammatory chemicals. In a recent study, one chiropractic treatment to the thoracic spine was shown to decrease blood plasma levels of pro-inflammatory chemicals (known as cytokines). (*Journal of Manipulative & Physiological Therapeutics*, Volume 29, Number 1; pages 14-21)

Research regarding the effects of chiropractic treatment is ongoing and promising. Currently, studies on disabling diseases such as asthma, multiple sclerosis, Alzheimer's, angina, and others are underway.

Although spinal manipulation is utilized by most chiropractors and is the treatment method most commonly associated with chiropractic, this mode of treatment is only one "arrow in the quiver" of the Doctor of Chiropractic. In my office, for example, a variety of patient and condition-specific methods of treatment are utilized to get the most relief and correction in the least amount of time.

Other commonly used treatment modalities by chiropractors include:

Disc Decompression Therapy

Flexion Distraction Disc Decompression therapy is a gentle, non-force technique used primarily for the treatment of spinal disc disorders (degenerative disc disease, annular tears, herniated and bulging discs, spinal stenosis, etc.). With this treatment approach, chiropractic providers use a specialized table that is designed to traction your spine while the doctor gently flexes you forward. When combined with decompression, flexion (bending forward) of the spine tends to open up the spinal canal and decrease nerve pressure.

Flexion distraction decompression therapy has been shown to

- Increase intervertebral disc height.
- Remove tension in the pain-sensitive outer annular fibers of the intervertebral disc.

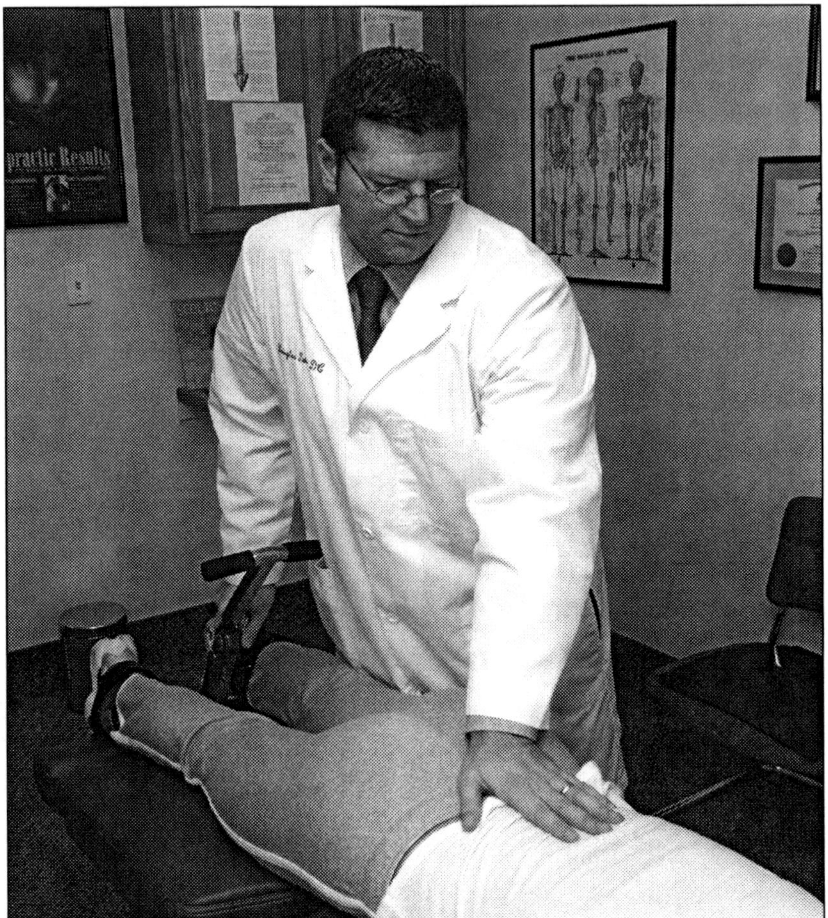

Dr. Taber performing flexion-distraction therapy.

• Decrease (drop) the pressure within the inside (nucleus) of the disc.

• Open up the intervertebral foramen where the spinal nerve exits.

• Restore motion to spinal joints.

In a 2005 study in the *European Spine Journal*, this technique was shown to be more effective than exercise for patients with low back pain and sciatica. In my office, this treatment is often combined with exercises and produces dramatic results.

In addition, there are multiple published case studies showing reduction of disc protrusions and herniations, decreased disc-related back and leg pain, and restoration of function with this technique.

Manual Soft Tissue Therapy

Manual (hands-on) therapy is a major focus of chiropractic care. Doctors of Chiropractic undergo a rigorous education in the evaluation and treatment of disorders associated with soft tissues.

Manual therapy is a general term that describes any treatment delivered by the hands. This includes trigger point therapy, strain-counterstrain, muscle energy techniques, joint mobilization, active release, and other forms of doctor-guided stretching and massage techniques.

In an article cited in a 2003 issue of *Spine*, manual (hands-on) therapy was shown to be more effective than exercise for chronic low back pain. Spinal pain specialists often utilize these treatments in acute or chronic cases where the soft tissue has become overly tight or fibrosis has set in.

Trigger Point Therapy

A trigger point is a highly irritable localized spot of tenderness in a nodule in a palpable taut band of muscle tissue. In short, this means that a trigger point is a 'knot' of muscle that you can feel with your fingers and hurts a lot when you press on it. A trigger point is a small patch of muscle in a state of continuous spasm that is very sore and which interferes with normal blood circulation and function of the whole muscle. Like a rubber band with a small section that has lost its elasticity and has instead become hardened and brittle, trigger points cause the muscle to be tight, stiff, weak and yet very tense at the same time. Trigger points are very sore to the touch, and they may feel like a thick band or knot that you can roll your fingers over.

Trigger points frequently form in injured muscles and can lead to a wide range of conditions, such as headaches, neck and shoulder pain, low back pain, arm and leg pain, as well as tennis elbow and carpal tunnel syndrome. They are the source of pain in many joints of the body such as the shoulder, wrist, hip, knee, and ankle and are often mistaken for arthritis, tendonitis, bursitis, or ligament injury. Trigger points frequently cause symptoms such as dizziness, earaches, nausea, heartburn, and numbness in the hands and feet. Even fibromyalgia may have its beginnings with trigger points. Some of the structural changes may be irreversible if trigger points are left untreated for long enough.

Trigger point therapy is a bodywork technique that involves the applying of pressure or ice massage to trigger points in order to relieve pain and dysfunction in other parts of the body. It is sometimes also called myofascial ("myo-" meaning muscle, "fascial" meaning connective tissue) trigger point therapy. Massage of the trigger point flushes the tissue and helps the trigger point's contracted sarcomeres to begin to release. In dealing directly with the trigger point, massage is the safest, most natural, and most effective form of pain therapy. To diffuse a trigger point, pressure is applied to the area for approximately 10 seconds, released, and then applied again for 10 more seconds in a pumping action while you breathe deeply.

After a series of treatments, circulation is restored, spasms disappear, irritation of the nerve endings in the muscle ceases, and the muscle is able to function normally again. As an added benefit, releasing trigger points also releases endorphins, which help to reduce stress and tension in other parts of the body.

Massage Therapy

Massage is the practice of applying pressure or vibration to the soft tissues of the body, including muscles, connective tissue, tendons, ligaments, and joints, and can be focused to specific parts of the body to heal injuries, or to the whole body to help relieve stress and tension. When most people think of massage, they think of a nice relaxing bodyworking that feels great and will help them become more relaxed. Unfortunately, for treating soft tissue injuries, this type of massage is not as useful as two other forms of massage – deep tissue massage and myofascial release.

Deep tissue massage techniques are generally designed for more focused massage work. Working a specific joint, muscle, or muscle group, the practitioner can access deeper layers of the soft tissue. Starting superficially and easing into the depth of the muscle slowly often allows more movement. This is the recommended approach in this modality since each person experiences pressure differently. If the pressure is applied too deeply or too quickly, the muscle may tighten to protect that area, and unnecessary damage or inflammation can be induced.

Myofascial release refers to the manual technique for stretching the fascia with the aim to balance the body. Fascia is located between the skin and the underlying structure of muscle and bone; it is a seamless web of connective tissue that covers and connects the muscles, organs, and skeletal structures in our body. Injuries, stress, trauma, and poor posture cause the fascia to become tight and inflamed. Because of the web-like structure of fascia, tightness in one part of the body can spread to other places in the body - much like pulling a thread in a piece of fabric. The goal of myofascial release is to release fascial restriction and restore its tissue.

Strain-Counterstrain

Strain-counterstrain technique, which I have been trained in and regularly use in my office, is aimed at painful "tender points" that have resulted in abnormal neuromuscular reflexes caused by structural and postural problems.

This technique is often useful in acute or extremely delicate situations. It involves finding the painful tender point and seeking a position of comfort until the tenderness diminishes. Then, a slow stretch is performed on the muscle, allowing it to reset to its normal level of tension and begin healing.

Physiotherapy

Chiropractors often use traditional physiotherapy modalities to assist in treatment to speed and enhance healing. Although useful in some situations (such as tendonitis and bursitis of elbows and shoulders), many of these modalities have not shown to be very effective for long-term (over 2-4 weeks) management of neck or back pain.

Ice Therapy

Ice has long been used to treat many painful conditions and is most often used to reduce swelling and help control pain immediately after an injury and throughout the inflammatory stage. When ice packs are applied, they can decrease the temperatures of the surrounding tissues by 10-15 degrees Fahrenheit, slowing down the metabolism in the tissues and reducing inflammation and pain.

Cold applied to the area decreases the flow of fluids into the tissues and slows the release of chemicals that cause pain and inflammation. Cold decreases feeling in an area by reducing the ability of the nerve endings to conduct impulses. The pain-relieving effect of ice results from decreased firing of the pain nerves and a relaxation of the muscle fibers. Cold also decreases the activity of cells, which works to reduce swelling and internal bleeding at the site of acute injury. Cooling the deep tissue also reduces muscle spasm by reducing the muscle's ability to maintain a contraction.

Heat Therapy

Heat therapy involves the application of hot packs to the surface of the skin in an effort to heat the underlying tissues. The warmth decreases muscle spasm, relaxes tense muscles, relieves pain, increases blood flow and can increase range of motion. However, because heat can also increase inflammation in an injured area, it is important to never use heat therapy during the initial acute stages of an injury when inflammation is at its worst.

Heat therapy is most effective when used in conjunction with an active exercise program and can be used effectively as part of a home care program under the supervision of a chiropractor.

Therapeutic Ultrasound

Therapeutic ultrasound is a form of deep heat therapy created by very high frequency sound waves, hence the name ultra-sound. These sound waves are a form of micro-massage

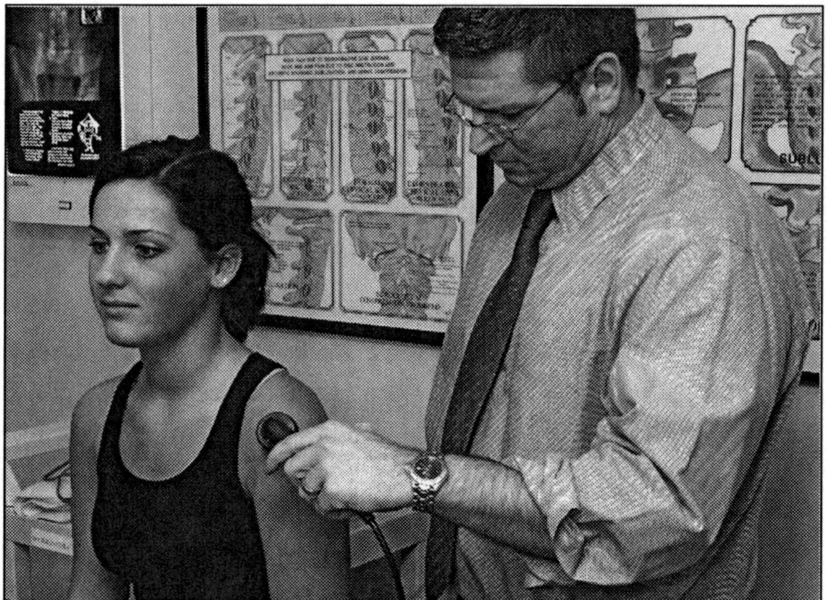

Therapeutic ultrasound is often useful in the management of injuries when combined with other physical treatment modalities. Back and neck injuries, as well as shoulder, hip, or elbow pain from bursitis and tendonitis are often treated successfully with this safe, painless procedure.

that help reduce swelling, increase blood flow, decrease pain, and speed healing. Ideally, ultrasound treatment should begin immediately after a trauma and may be administered daily. It has been shown to reduce the inflammatory period and thereby accelerate the healing process. During the repair stage, ultrasound can stimulate the development of the capillaries necessary to re-establish a healthy blood supply to the damaged area.

One of the greatest benefits of ultrasound is in the later stages of healing where the primary goal of therapy is to increase soft tissue flexibility. The deep heating effects of ultrasound make the muscles more pliable and, when combined with stretching, ultrasound is very useful for increasing the range of motion in the neck and upper back.

In 2001, the results of a study comparing spinal manipulation to ultrasound was presented at the 4th Interdisciplinary World Congress on Low Back and Pelvic Pain. This randomized, controlled trial compared the two treatments on 46 men and 66 women with low back pain for at least 3 months. The conclusion was clear: spinal manipulation is more effective than ultrasound therapy for chronic low back pain.

Electric Muscle Stimulation

Electrical stimulation dates all the way back to the ancient Egyptian doctors, who held electric eels against the body of their patients to help alleviate headaches. Today, there are a number of different electrical stimulation (EMS) therapies available, all with their own particular benefits. Some are more beneficial for pain relief or to reduce inflammation, some for muscle spasm, and some actually cause muscles to contract in order to reduce muscle atrophy. In general, this type of therapy transmits light electrical pulses through the skin and into specific areas of the body.

Interferential therapy is a unique type of electrical stimulation that is very effective in decreasing pain and muscle spasm, and is very helpful during healing. One of the greatest benefits of interferential therapy is its ability to prevent the development of myofascial pain syndromes during the initial stages of healing after an injury when the muscles are the most vulnerable. It can be useful in promoting soft tissue healing and the restoration of muscle strength. The use of interferential therapy can dramatically improve the rate and degree of recovery and is often used in our clinic for acute pain.

Cervical Spine Traction

Chiropractors often use traction of the cervical spine (neck) to decompress tight muscles and open up the space around pinched nerves. Although this should be avoided in some cases, such as an unstable neck or severe bony spurs, many patients feel relief with just a few traction treatments. In some cases, a home traction device will be prescribed by your doctor so you may enjoy the benefits without a visit to the office.

According to a 2002 article in *Neurosurgical Focus*, 75% of patients with neck and arm pain, muscle weakness, and loss of a reflex will respond to traction of the neck. Another 2002 article, this one in the medical publication *Radiology*, studied what happens to a cervical disc herniation during traction. The patients underwent an MRI while traction was applied to their neck. Eighteen of the twenty-one patients studied had partial reduction of their herniations, and three actually had complete resolution!

Exercise

No treatment program for pain is complete without involvement of the patient in his or her care. Although many therapies are passive (administered to you by a doctor or therapist), it is the active (patient-guided) tools that cannot be neglected or underemphasized. The success or failure in correcting a spinal problem rests largely on your determination to play an active role in your care.

Because of its safety and effectiveness when used appropriately, exercise is a main area of focus in most chiropractic offices. I spend a great deal of time designing exercise programs, explaining exercise techniques, and guiding patients through rehab programs.

Exercise and rehabilitation programs should not be "cookie cutter;" every patient is different. Your specific condition, level of fitness, areas of improper function or deconditioning, and other factors need to be considered when your doctor or therapist prescribes an exercise program for you.

For example, as a former Personal Trainer, often many patients ask me to provide them with a strengthening program using weights or machines to perform at the gym in order to

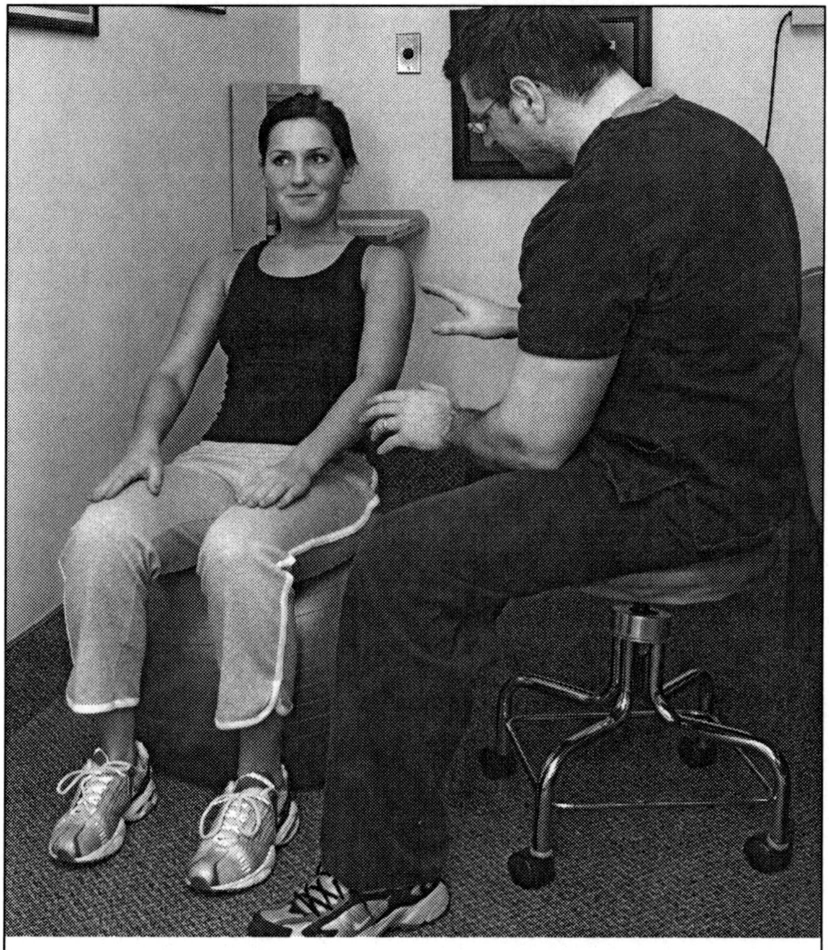

Rehabilitation is important for preventing re-injury and is a main focus of chiropractic care once a condition has stabilized.

make their back stronger after an injury. Their train of thought is that some type of weakness in the large muscles of their back is responsible for causing pain. Often, however, weakness in the spinal muscles is not the issue. Rather, weak abdominal muscles, deep spinal muscles that rotate or flex the spine, or an imbalance between the spinal and abdominal muscles is the problem. For such patients, stronger abdominal muscles or a core stability program will offer a better outcome than a strengthening program of weight lifting for the extensor muscles in the back.

Another example, The McKenzie Method, is an exercise protocol commonly prescribed for patients with low back pain and tends to emphasize extension (bending backwards) as part of the routine. Although effective for many types of back pain, these exercises may not be recommended for people with spinal stenosis, spondylolisthesis, and certain facet syndromes.

The wrong type of exercises or program can prolong recovery or even increase the risk of injury. Doctors of Chiropractic are well trained in detecting muscular weakness and patterns of imbalance in the human body, and many chiropractors have extensive experience and post-graduate training in McKenzie Therapy, Williams Flexion Protocols, Spinal Core Stability & Multifidus exercises or other forms of spinal exercise and rehabilitation therapy.

Remember, every treatment protocol for back or neck pain should have some type of exercise component. Some basic exercises that may help in preventing back and neck pain, known as Prehab (preventative rehabilitation) exercises are presented in Chapter 10. For a more detailed or thorough program, seek care with your Doctor of Chiropractic.

Proprioceptive Taping

Proprioception refers to the body's ability to sense movement within joints enabling you to know where our limbs are in space without having to look. The proprioceptive system is made up of special nerves in the muscles, joints, and ligaments that can sense tension and stretch and pass this information to the brain.

When a part of the body is injured, there is often a disruption in the proprioceptive system, resulting in a loss of normal sensation and coordinated movement. This can leave you prone to re-injury and decrease your performance if you are involved in a sport.

One simple way of re-establishing normal proprioception in a damaged area of the body is with proprioceptive taping. Proprioceptive taping involves placing strips of tape across an injured area in an attempt to brace or overstimulate the nerves in the area. This allows the brain and nervous system to develop normal coordination and restore function.

Spinal Pelvic Stabilizer Orthotics

Because we consider ourselves "architects of the spine," many chiropractors prescribe foot orthotics for patients. In cases where there is a leg length discrepancy or foot disorder contributing to altered biomechanics in the pelvis and spine, orthotics play a role in stabilizing the region "from the ground up."

Results from a 2003 pilot study suggest that custom-made Spinal Pelvic Stabilizers help improve body balance while standing. Studies in 1996 and 2002 in *The Journal of Manipulative & Physiological Therapeutics* and *The Journal of Sports Chiropractic and Rehabilitation* have shown that Spinal Pelvic Stabilizers from the Foot Levelers company may help improve alignment, function, performance, and gait (walking).

Nutritional Support

Proper nutrition is vital during the process of healing and recovering from an injury. In addition, many recent dietary recommendations and nutritional supplements may decrease inflammation or slow the progression of degenerative spinal disorders. Doctors of Chiropractic are one of the few health care providers who stress nutrition and diet in treating and preventing disease. We will discuss nutrition in more detail in Chapter 11.

Medication Assisted Manual Therapy

Medication Assisted Manual Therapy (MAMT) is a new frontier in the effort to treat chronic pain. As the name implies, this treatment involves a combination of various medications and anesthesia combined with manipulation. This approach requires a team effort of medical doctors and chiropractors and is often administered in hospitals or ambulatory surgical centers such as the Binghamton Spine Care Center.

Manipulation Under Joint Anesthesia (MUJA), Manipulation Post-Epidural Steroid Injection (MPESI), and Manipulation Under Anesthesia (MUA) are three procedures that fall under this category. These procedures are discussed further in Chapter 9.

The Three Phases of Chiropractic Care

Chiropractic care following an injury is like building a house – certain things have to happen in a particular order for everything to stand. When building a house, if you tried to put up your walls before you had a solid foundation, your walls would be weak and eventually collapse. If you tried to put on your roof before the walls were ready, you would run into the same problem. The same is true for your body, which has to go through a particular plan of care in order to repair itself correctly and fully. There are three general phases of chiropractic care: 1) relief care, 2) corrective care, and 3) maintenance care. How long each phase of care takes depends on the severity of your injuries.

Phase One - Relief Care

Many people go to a chiropractor because they are in pain. In this first phase of care, the main goal is to relieve you of your symptoms. Sometimes this will require frequent treatments.

The Three Phases of Chiropractic Care

PHASE 1	PHASE 2	PHASE 3
Relief Care	Corrective Care	Maintenance Care
If you are in pain when you come to our office, the first objective is to help you feel better.	*During the corrective care phase, muscles and other tissues are allowed to heal more completely, thereby helping prevent re-injury.*	*Once your body has fully healed, it is important to come in for periodic adjustments to avoid problems in the future.*
Depending on the severity of your problem, it is typical to be treated 2-3 times per week for 4-12 weeks.	*It is typical to be treated 2-4 times per month for 6-24 months, depending on your overall health and the severity of your problem.*	*Usually, this only requires a quick visit to the chiropractor about once a month or so.*

Most people are under the assumption that if they don't feel any pain that there is nothing wrong with them – that they are healthy. Unfortunately, pain is a very poor indicator of health. In fact, pain and other symptoms frequently only appear after a disease or other condition has become advanced. For example, consider a cavity in your tooth. Does it hurt when it first develops or only after it has become serious? How about heart disease? Regardless of whether you are talking about cancer, heart disease, diabetes, stress, or problems with the spine, pain is usually the last thing to appear. When you begin chiropractic care, pain is also the first symptom to disappear, even though much of the underlying condition remains.

Phase Two - Corrective Care

Most chiropractors regard the elimination of symptoms as the easiest part of a course of treatment. If all that the chiropractor does is to remove the pain and stop there, the chances of the condition recurring are much greater. In order to avoid

Dramatic Results from Chiropractic Care

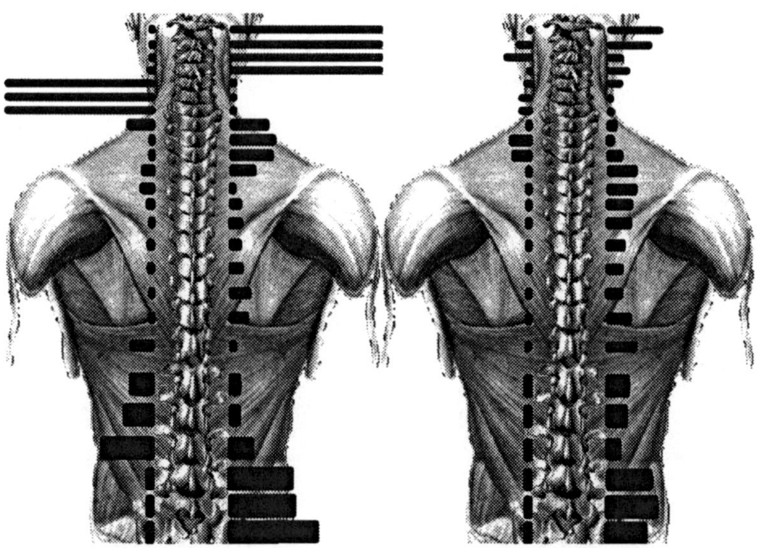

Before *After Six Months of Care*

In these thermal scans of the spine, a definite improvement is seen after six months of chiropractic care. In the "before" image, there were several areas that were very inflamed, indicated by the long bars. In the "after" image, the shorter bars indicate a substantial decrease of irritation and inflammation in the spine. This particular patient had been suffering from neck and low back pain for several years before seeking care. When the first scan was made, she had extreme neck and low back pain. At the time of the second scan, she was pain-free.

a rapid recurrence of symptoms, it may be necessary to continue treatment even though your symptoms are gone.

During the correction phase of your treatment, you will not have to be treated as often as you did during the first phase of care and, depending on your particular circumstances, you may begin doing exercises and stretches at home to help accelerate your healing. Do not be discouraged if you have mild flare-ups in your symptoms on occasion; this is normal. Flare-ups are bound to occur during the corrective phase because your body has not fully recovered. Depending on the severity of your injury or condition and how long you have been suffering from it, this phase of your care may last anywhere from a few weeks to several months.

Phase Three - Maintenance Care

Once your body has fully healed, routine maintenance chiropractic care can help ensure that your physical problems do not return, and keep your body in optimal condition. Just like continuing an exercise program and eating well in order to sustain the benefits of exercise and proper diet, it is necessary to continue chiropractic care to ensure the health of your musculoskeletal system. When you make routine chiropractic care a part of your lifestyle, you can avoid many of the aches and pains that so many people suffer.

8

Frequently Asked Questions

"Seize the moment of excited curiosity on any subject to solve your doubts. If you let it pass, the desire may neve return, and you may remain in ignorance."

- William Wirt 1772-1834

Q: Are chiropractors real doctors?

Chiropractors are licensed as medical health care providers in every U.S. state and dozens of countries around the world. While the competition to attend chiropractic school is not as fierce as medical school, the chiropractic and medical school curricula are virtually identical. In fact, chiropractors have more hours of education than their medical counterparts. As part of their education, chiropractic students also complete approximately nine hundred hours of work in a clinical setting, assisting licensed chiropractors. Once chiropractic students graduate, they have to pass four sets of national board exams as well as state board exams in the states they want to practice.

Chiropractors receive extensive training, combined with many hours of practical work. Just like conventional medical doctors, chiropractors are medical professionals that are subject to the same testing, licensing, and monitoring by state and national peer-reviewed boards. Federal and state programs, such as Medicare and Workers' Compensation programs, cover chiropractic, and all federal agencies accept sick-leave certificates signed by Doctors of Chiropractic.

The biggest difference between chiropractors and medical doctors lies not in their education or diagnostic ability but in their preferred method of treatment. Medical doctors are trained in the use of medications (chemicals that affect your internal biochemistry) and surgery. Consequently, if you have a chemical problem such as diabetes, hypothyroidism, or an infection, medical doctors can be very helpful. However, if your problem is mechanical or physical, there is no chemical in existence that can fix it. You need a physical treatment to correct a physical problem. That's where chiropractic care is at the forefront. Chiropractors use physical treatments – adjustments, exercises, stretches, physiotherapies – to treat conditions that are physical, rather than chemical, in origin such as back pain, injuries, disc problems, muscle spasms, headaches, and poor posture.

Chiropractic Education

Subject	Chiropractic Schools Total Hours	Medical Schools Total Hours
Anatomy	456	215
Biochemistry	161	100
Microbiology	145	145
Neurology	149	171
Physiology	243	174
Pathology	296	507
Psychology	56	323
Radiology	271	13
Orthopedics	168	2
Diagnosis	408	113
Obstetrics / Gynecology	66	284
Total Hours	**2,419**	**2,047**

(Based on the average the curriculum of 18 chiropractic colleges and 22 medical schools)

Q: Do chiropractors work with medical doctors?

Absolutely. At my office, I work hand in hand with medical professionals everyday. Personally, I enjoy working with primary care physicians, pain specialists, and spine surgeons in an attempt to get the best outcome for my patients.

I communicate regularly with medical doctors, both to keep them informed on the status of their patient, and to offer my input on difficult cases. Patients benefit when there is open communication between health care providers, and this is encouraged in my office.

A recent survey of 15,000 Harvard Medical School faculty, published in the *Harvard Health Letter*, revealed that 13% of the physicians have had chiropractic treatment. That is 50-75% more than the national average of Americans who seek chiropractic care.

When a doctor refers a patient to my office for care, I take the trust they have placed in me by sending their patient to be both a great compliment and responsibility.

Q: How do I find the right chiropractor?

Finding a good chiropractor can be difficult, because the chiropractic profession has an unusually large variety of practice philosophies. It is often useful to ask friends, co-workers, and neighbors for their recommendations. Primary care physicians or other health care providers may also be helpful. Generally speaking, if many resources recommend the same chiropractor, there's a good chance that he or she is reputable.

General questions that you may want to ask when seeking a Doctor of Chiropractic include

- Does the doctor have a bachelors' degree as well as a doctoral degree?

- Have they completed the National Boards?
- How many years have they been in practice?
- Do they require x-rays before treatment?
- Will the doctor stay in communication with my other health care providers?
- Do they belong to any reputable associations, academies, or societies?
- Does the doctor have post-graduate training or advanced certification in any specific treatment technique or method?

Although it is a common question, whether or not a chiropractor takes your insurance often has little to do with their experience or training. Many highly qualified chiropractors accept insurance coverage, but just as many doctors prefer to steer clear of the managed care system.

Be wary of "Free Consultations," "Free X-Rays," "New Patient Dinners," or other advertising gimmicks that some doctors use to attract new patients. Clinical examinations and x-ray imaging are diagnostic tests, not marketing tools.

Avoid doctors who recommend lengthy (more than 3-4 months) pre-scheduled treatment plans. This approach often requires pre-payment up front, and the care plan usually has little or no rhyme or reason. Every patient is different, and no doctor can predict how much treatment you will require in a year. Many patients do require extensive chiropractic care, but this is a decision that must be made as the care progresses, not at the first visit or several months in advance.

Q: What is a chiropractic adjustment?

The chiropractic adjustment is a gentle, quick thrust to a particular joint, typically in the spine, intended to restore normal position and movement. Adjustments are important for releasing adhesions in the joint and reducing stress on the nervous system. Because of the fact that the nervous system is the master controller of all muscles and organs in the body, removing stress on the nervous system through chiropractic adjustments will frequently lead to improved health in the entire body.

Q: Do chiropractic adjustments hurt? Are there side effects from using chiropractic for treating back pain?

Usually not. There have been some patients of mine who have experienced mild soreness after being adjusted, but this is more of the exception. Most people feel better very quickly after being adjusted.

Patients may or may not experience side effects from chiropractic treatment. Effects may include temporary discomfort in parts of the body that were treated, headache, or tiredness. These effects tend to be minor and resolve within 1 to 2 days.

Q: How many adjustments will I need?

The number of manipulation treatments you will need depends on several factors including 1) your age, 2) your overall health, 3) the extent of degenerative changes, de-conditioning, or spinal distortion.

If you are young, in good health, and have a mild condition that occurred very recently, you will need far fewer adjustments than if you are older, in poor general health, and have been struggling with a problem for many years. The total number of adjustments you will need also depends on whether you are merely interested in reducing the pain you are currently experiencing, or are interested in creating optimal long-term health.

Q: Do I have to undergo x-rays to see a chiropractor?

Although x-rays are often useful for chiropractors, they are not always necessary. Chiropractors, like any doctor, only order tests when they feel that the results of these tests will give useful information in the diagnosis of what is wrong with the patient. Established guidelines and clinical experience are used in determining whether or not x-rays will be useful in any particular case. Be wary of any practitioner who requires x-rays before treatment or orders repeated x-rays of the same region of your spine to assess your progress.

Q: My friend is a physical therapist, and he says that he performs spinal manipulation. Isn't that the same as a chiropractic treatment?

In a word, no. I have tremendous respect for the profession of physical therapy. I have had the opportunity to work with some of whom I consider the best PT's in the nation. I have taken classes and seminars with physical therapists. I frequently recommend physical therapy for patients who have suffered a knee injury, rotator cuff tear, or ankle sprain. When I feel that my patients require a supervised exercise program or the use of weight training machines, I recommend that they go to a physical therapist for consultation.

However, when it comes to the treatment of spine-related pain syndromes and hands-on manipulation of the spinal joints, chiropractors have extensive, specific training that qualifies them as the spinal care specialists.

Over ninety percent of spinal manipulation is performed by Doctors of Chiropractic. Chiropractors have advanced training in diagnosis, evaluation, articular neurology, biomechanics, and other areas pertaining to spinal pain syndromes.

Because recent studies have shown this treatment to be effective for a variety of conditions, many non-chiropractic practitioners are trying to use spinal manipulation in their practice. The limited use of physiotherapy modalities (ultrasound, electric muscle simulation, etc.) for back pain, especially chronic back pain, has prompted therapists (physical, occupation, and massage) as well as some medical doctors to pursue "crash courses" on spinal manipulation. They may attend classes or weekend courses to learn how to perform spinal manipulation, and then use their limited knowledge of technique to "adjust" their patients. In my opinion, this is dangerous and inappropriate from a clinical standpoint.

When my patients require surgery, I send them to a board certified surgeon. Although I understand, have observed, and have read about what surgical techniques and options are out there, I do not have the training or expertise to wield the scalpel. I would never think of it, because my training lies elsewhere. This is precisely why, when patients have spinal syndromes that are best treated with various forms of manual (hands-on) therapy and spinal manipulation techniques, it is best left to the experts in the delivery of these procedures – a qualified Doctor of Chiropractic.

In 2000, the Department of Health & Human Services echoed this sentiment and concern for patient safety when they issued the statute (Section 1861r of the Social Security Act) stating that non-physician physical therapists may not perform manual manipulation to correct a vertebral subluxation.

In addition to therapeutic goals, there are dangerous diagnostic limitations. If a patient presents with low back pain to a PT without a referral from their doctor or chiropractor, and there is some question as to what is causing the pain, how will the therapist find out?

PT's are not physicians, and, although many have taken post-graduate courses and attained Doctor of Physical Therapy

(DPT) degrees in an attempt to gain direct access to patients (rather than through the referral of a physician), they still lack the training and licensure necessary to order important diagnostic tests.

The danger of direct access for physical therapists is not lost on the medical community. John S. Gould, M.D. in the March 2005 issue of *The American Journal of Orthopedics*, states, "For a patient to make his or her own diagnosis and try therapy directly…is to invite potential disaster: missed diagnosis, delayed treatment for non-mechanical disease, permanent injuries, and even death for the unwary patient. Unwary patients should not be relegated to the care of individuals who…have clearly limited medical knowledge and skills and may not know their real limitations."

It has been said that specialists know more about less. In the area of spine care, and especially spinal manipulation, Doctors of Chiropractic are the safest and most effective choice.

Q: I have heard that chiropractic neck adjustments will cause you to have a stroke. Is this true?

Strokes are definitely serious events, no doubt, and there are some medical doctors who still tell their patients to avoid going to the chiropractor because sooner or later, they say, adjustments of the neck will cause a stroke. There is no denying that a possibility of this happening exists. However, the risk of suffering a stroke from a chiropractic adjustment is extremely small, about the risk of being struck by lightning. In fact, you are 70,000 times more likely to suffer a stroke from the daily use of aspirin to prevent heart attacks than to suffer a stroke from a chiropractic adjustment. You are 37,000 times more likely to suffer a stroke for an unknown reason than to suffer a stroke from a chiropractic adjustment. When administered by a licensed doctor of chiropractic, adjustments are extremely safe.

Statistically, the likelihood of a vertebral artery dissection (which can result in a stroke) is estimated to be 1 in 500,000 to 1 in 300,000. These complication rates are considerably less than any treatment modality (even an aspirin) for spinal pain management.

The risk of suffering a fatal stroke from a manipulation of the neck is 0.00025%. The risk of having a stroke in the general public is 0.00057%. What does this mean? The risk of having a stroke "out of the blue" is higher than the risk associated with a stroke from a manipulation of the neck.

Doctors of Chiropractic are trained to diagnose patients who may be prone to this disorder and may order tests to rule out the risk of stroke. When there may be a risk of vascular problems, chiropractic techniques are changed or modified to avoid such complications.

Q: My insurance company covers chiropractic care, but the number of visits is limited. Why?

How many Tylenol will you take this year? How many times will you slip or fall? How many times will you need to exercise or eat right to maintain a level of health? Can you honestly predict in advance what the next 365 days may hold in store? I cannot predict in advance how many of any treatment a patient will need in a one-year period, so I don't know how insurance companies do it.

Many patients in my office are just fine after 1-2 treatments. Minor sprains or strains rarely involve an extensive treatment program. As I mentioned in the introduction, my first experience with chiropractic, at the age of 22 with a low back sprain, involved only one treatment session.

However, patients with advanced degenerative changes, spinal deformities, congenital anomalies, or disc disorders often require more extensive chiropractic treatment. Patients with disc disorders in the neck or low back may require 6-12 weeks of treatment, and sometimes more, to minimize the risk of nerve damage and postpone or prevent surgery. For some reason, however, this fact eludes insurance companies who "ration" medical and chiropractic treatment to their consumers (also known as patients) in an attempt to cut costs and appease company stockholders.

In my opinion, the determination of the number or frequency of treatments should be left to the discretion of the treating doctor and is not the same for everyone. In addition, my opinion is that supportive or maintenance chiropractic care as a means of preventing recurrence of symptoms and restoration of function is a patient and doctor-based decision, and should not be left to the discretion of an insurance carrier, whose primary interest is cost containment.

Currently, there are multiple class action suits against insurance companies who have allegedly limited care or denied appropriate tests and medically necessary treatment for patients. If you allow insurance companies to dictate your access to health and wellness, you are leaving yourself in the wrong hands. I personally have been asked to sit in with insurance companies, and the ways in which they make their decisions and protocols can be scary.

In the 21st century, doctors find themselves in a compromising position. Managed (or "mangled") care has put a tremendous strain on the practice of every form of medicine.

As cited in Dr. Terry Rondberg's book, Under The Influence of Modern Medicine, a 1997 article in *The Journal of the American Medical Association* accurately predicted what the commercialization of medicine (also known as managed care) carries with it. A list of potential hazards with managed care includes

Diversion of funds. When a portion of funds for care for the sick and injured are diverted for corporate objectives (stockholder dividends, advertising, executive salaries, etc.), resources available for health care are reduced. (note: Have you ever seen those sharp pens or clipboards with your insurance company's logo on them? Guess how they were paid for.)

Risk avoidance. Excluding people from coverage because of prior disease, genetics, predisposition, or high cost denies care to those most in need.

Downgrading personnel. Highly qualified but expensive personnel will be threatened by discharge in favor of others with less experience and fewer credentials but lower income expectations.

Monopoly and loss of freedom of choice. Smaller communities, rural America, and the inner city are often areas where the population and financial resources are not sufficient enough to attract choices for health care insurances. This often results in less freedom for people to choose the best insurance plan for their situation.

Managed care has infiltrated the daily practice of medicine. For example, more often than not, doctors are forced to request authorization for tests such as x-rays and MRI's from an insurance company before they may order them. I do this almost daily, and it is both time consuming and humiliating.

What does the clinical research say about managed care and chiropractic costs?

According to a 1998 article in *The Spine Journal*, chiropractic care represents 2.9% of all costs associated with treating low back pain. Physical therapy costs were 20%, and surgery represented 21% of these costs.

In 2003, a study in *The Journal of Manipulative & Physiological Therapeutics* revealed that chiropractic care reduces hospital admissions for back pain by 43%, reduces outpatient surgeries by 43.2%, and decreases the cost of prescription medication by 51.8%.

A similar study, published in the October 11th, 2004 issue of *The Archives of Internal Medicine*, showed that chiropractic care decreased the cost of treating back pain by 28%, with a reduction of 41% in hospitalization and a 32% decrease in the need for surgery.

In 1992, the Bureau of Disability Economics Research at the University of Richmond concluded that chiropractic costs for treatment of arthritis and low back pain, including disc disorders, is lower than the cost of medical care.

The Manga Report on The Effectiveness and Cost Effectiveness of Chiropractic Management of Low Back Pain, stated in 1992 that, "There would be highly significant cost savings if more management of low back pain was transferred from physicians to chiropractors…users of chiropractic care have substantially lower health care costs, especially inpatient costs, than those treated with medical care only."

According to a 1988 study of 10,652 low back cases in the Florida Workers' Compensation System, the duration of total disability was 51.3% less for chiropractic patients. The cost of treating these patients with chiropractic was 58.5% lower than medical care, and only 20.3% of chiropractic patients were hospitalized (versus 52.2% of medical patients.) (Wolk S: Chiropractic vs. Medical Care: A cost analysis of disability and treatment for back related Worker's Compensation cases.)

A 1988 study conducted by the Utah Workers' Compensation Board, and published in *The Journal of Occupational Medicine* (1991;33:847-52) found that the mean compensation cost paid for patients under medical care for low back pain was $668.39, while the mean cost paid for chiropractic patients was $68.38.

These studies, and several others, have clearly shown that chiropractic care

- represents a fraction of health care costs
- is effective in reducing hospitalization
- results in less disability
- minimizes the need for surgery
- decreases the use of prescription drugs, and
- returns people to work faster

I would say that's a pretty good track record for any healthcare discipline, and certainly does not warrant arbitrary limits on care.

The next time you ask yourself why certain types of treatment are restricted or denied by your insurance company, consider a 2002 article in The Journal of the American Medical Association, which stated that "59% of the experts who write clinical guidelines that define good medical care have direct financial ties to the companies whose services are being offered."

Bear in mind that medicine, chiropractic or otherwise, is an art, philosophy, and science. Every patient is different, and when the art of practicing medicine is dictated by insurance bureaucracy or arbitrary care restrictions, your doctor's structured and rational decision-making process, and maybe your health, is being compromised.

Q: Can pregnant women undergo chiropractic care?

Chiropractic care is a safe and effective treatment for back pain during pregnancy. Low back pain is common during pregnancy, affecting over 60% of pregnant women. Expecting women are referred to my office almost weekly by their OB/GYN or midwife for problems in the low back, pelvis, or legs. Because they must avoid many medications for the sake of a healthy baby, many women seek natural methods of care for their problem.

A January, 2006, article in the *Journal of Midwifery and Women's Health*, reported that chiropractic treatment is safe (no adverse effects were seen in the 17 cases studied) and effective in reducing pain intensity associated with pregnancy.

Q: Do Doctors of Chiropractic prescribe medication?

Currently, chiropractors do not prescribe medications, although they may refer someone to another provider for prescription medication if it is deemed necessary. In most cases, however, patients are better off with physical, rather than chemical, treatments for physical problems.

We know that a chiropractic adjustment is safer than taking an aspirin. We also know that masking symptoms with drugs usually does nothing to actually solve the underlying problem, and that long-term use of narcotic pain medications carries with it the potential to cause addiction and drug dependence.

I am far from "anti-medication." I personally believe that there are times when medication has short-term use in managing back pain. Studies suggest that acute bouts of back pain can be treated with a few days of medication in addition to conservative treatments. However, long term medication use for controlling back pain can be dangerous.

Q: I have read interviews with professional athletes and movie stars, and they often credit their chiropractor for their performance. Is this common?

A short list of the many movie stars and professional athletes that benefit from chiropractic care includes Tiger Woods, Lance Armstrong, Barry Bonds, Michael Jordan, Wayne Gretzky, Jerome Bettis, Mel Gibson, Sylvester Stallone, Robin Williams, Denzel Washington, Christie Brinkley, Arnold Schwarzenegger, Clint Eastwood, Jerry Seinfeld, Richard Gere, Muhammed Ali, Phil Collins, Steven Segal, Anthony Robbins, Nolan Ryan, and Fred Funk.

If top athletes and celebrities, who have to be in peak physical state in order to earn a living, benefit from chiropractic care, there must be something to its positive effects.

Q: Why is routine chiropractic care so important?

Many health-conscious adults go to the chiropractor for overall wellness and preventative measures. Chiropractic was originally founded on the premise that a properly functioning nervous system (for which the spine is the conduit from the brain to every organ and cell in the body) is vital for the expression of health.

Dr. Christopher Kent, in his testimony before the Senate Appropriations Committee, cited an insurance database analysis comparing chiropractic patients over 75 years old with patients of the same age who weren't seeing chiropractors. The data presented showed that the chiropractic patients reported better overall health, spent fewer days in nursing homes, used fewer prescription drugs, and were more active than the group of non-chiropractic patients.

In 1999, the *New England Journal of Medicine* shows us that chiropractic patients use 56% fewer anti-inflammatory drugs, 75% fewer muscle relaxants, and 98% less physical therapy in the management of their pain.

In 2000, a survey of 311 chiropractic patients, aged 65 and older, who had received chiropractic maintenance care for at least five years was reported in *The Journal of Manipulative & Physiological Therapeutics*. These patients, compared to those not undergoing chiropractic care, spent 31% less than the national average for health care costs. They saw health care providers, on an average, half as often. They used less prescription drugs and less tobacco than their non-chiropractic counterparts.

In 2004, a health survey of 2,818 chiropractic patients from 156 clinics was published in *The Journal of Alternative & Complementary Medicine*. This survey revealed that 95% of patients felt that their expectations had been met under chiropractic care, and 99% wished to continue care. In addition, there was a strong correlation between persons receiving chiropractic care and self-reported improvements in health, wellness, and quality of life.

As previously mentioned, research into the effects of chiropractic care beyond that of back pain is ongoing. Clinical trials have showed promising results in other areas, and Doctors of Chiropractic have long been advocates for a Wellness Lifestyle, addressing such factors as diet, emotional well-being, rest, nutrition, and exercise.

Q: Will I need to continue to see my chiropractor after my symptoms are gone?

How long you decide to benefit from chiropractic care is always up to you. As I have stated previously, many conditions respond quickly and require minimal care programs and in-office protocols. There is, however, mounting evidence that preventative or maintenance care is effective in some cases.

For example, in 2004, a study in the *Journal of Manipulative & Physiological Therapeutics* sought out to determine whether or not chiropractic care is able to actually prevent back pain flare-ups.

The authors studied 30 patients who suffered from back pain for at least 6 months. All patients underwent 12 chiropractic treatments over the course of one month. Then, half of the patients did not undergo any further chiropractic care for 9 months, while the other half continued chiropractic care once every three weeks for the nine-month period.

At the end of the nine-month period, both groups were examined again. The authors found that both groups had a reduction in their pain during the entire study period. However, the patients undergoing chiropractic care experienced a significantly greater reduction in disability than the patients who did not continue care.

Q: Has chiropractic care been compared to other treatments for back pain in any scientific studies or research?

There is a wealth of research that supports chiropractic care for a variety of conditions. Several studies have compared chiropractic to other common treatment methods.

In a 2004 survey by the U.S. Centers for Disease Control and Prevention, it was found that nearly 2/3 of Americans use alternative health care, with chiropractors being the most common.

Remember, chiropractors do not prescribe medication, so there is no funding from pharmaceutical companies or health care conglomerates. Chiropractic care has flourished because of results rather than political lobbying and mass marketing and advertising campaigns.

In an answer to the need for evidence-based treatment, chiropractic colleges, practitioners, insurance organizations, and even the federally funded National Institute for Health have intensively studied chiropractic treatment for modern health problems.

Here are just a few samples of the conclusions reached through extensive research on the effectiveness of chiropractic care compared to other treatments:

• For chronic back pain, chiropractic care has been shown to be more effective than acupuncture or anti-inflammatory drugs. (*Journal of Manipulative & Physiological Therapeutics*, 1999; 22:6. pages 376-381)

• In patients with chronic back pain, spinal maniplation results in greater short-term improvement than acupuncture or medication. (*Spine,* 2003 28: pages 1490-1503)

• Spinal manipulation has real benefits in patients with acute and chronic low back pain. (*The American Family Physician*, February 1, 2004)

• Chiropractic treatments are more beneficial than muscle relaxants in reducing the severity of patients' pain. (*Journal of Manipulative & Physiological Therapeutics*, 2004)

• Spinal manipulation provides greater improvement in symptoms, as well as greater improvement in function, for patients with back and neck pain compared to physical therapy. (*British Medical Journal*, 1992, pages 601-605)

• Chiropractic is more effective than hospital outpatient treatment for low back pain. (*British Medical Journal*,1990, pages 1431-1437)

• Chiropractic treatment (spinal manipulation) results in quicker pain relief and greater back mobility at two weeks than massage therapy. (*Manual Medicine*,1986, pages 68-71, and *Spine*, 1984, pages 301-304)

• Spinal manipulation provided significant improvement compared with codeine. (*Rheumatology & Rehabilitation*, 1978, pages 46-53)

9

Integrated Spine Care and Medical Therapies

*"If you focus on results, you will never see change.
If you focus on change, you will get results."*

- Jack Dixon

Integrated Spine Care: The Future of Back Pain Treatment

When spine specialists (chiropractors, spine surgeons, pain management specialists, physical therapists, etc.) work together, patients are privy to an integrated continuum of spine care that minimizes variability. In addition, this team approach to patient care minimizes "doctor hopping," which is a term that describes the repeated and often needless and expensive habit of going from one specialist to another in an attempt to find the magic pill or answer.

I have the unique opportunity to be Director of Conservative Care at a multidisciplinary spine care center in the Southern Tier of New York. In this setting, I work in tandem with spine specialists in the areas of surgery and spinal injections.

Difficult cases are often referred to our spine center by chiropractors and medical doctors with the hope that we may have something to offer that traditional therapies have not. When conservative care has been exhausted, our spine surgeons are confident that they are performing surgery on the right patients for the right reasons.

When specialists work together for the common goal of relieving patients' pain and returning them to normal function, there is less confusion for the patient and health care providers involved in the case. The need for such an approach was emphasized in a 2003 article in *The American Journal of Pain Management,* which recommends a "more seamless, coordinated approach to back pain care." This sentiment is echoed in various spine care studies and publications, and is being realized in integrated care centers such as the Texas Back Institute and the Binghamton Spine Care Center.

Severe cases of low back pain often require more aggressive therapy than simply oral medications. In these cases, there are several options available to help you eliminate your low back pain, such as trigger point and epidural injections, nerve blocks, facet blocks, and, if necessary, surgery.

Facet Blocks

Most back pain related to facet joints can be treated successfully with a combination of exercise, manipulation, and improved posture. When these are not enough to alleviate your pain, however, you may need an injection called a facet block. As you read earlier, the facet joints are paired joints in the back that have opposing surfaces of cartilage, and there is a capsule surrounding the entire joint. Twisting injuries to the spine can cause damage to one or both facet joints, causing pain. In cases where the facet joint itself is the pain generator, a facet block injection can be performed to alleviate the pain. Facet block injections are both diagnostic tools used to confirm the specific source of back pain as well as a therapy to decrease pain and inflammation in the joint.

In a facet block procedure, fluoroscopy (live x-ray) is used to guide the needle into the specific facet joint capsule to inject lidocaine (a numbing agent) and/or a steroid (an anti-inflammatory medication). If your pain goes away after the injection, it can confirm that the source of pain is the specific facet joint capsule that has just been injected.

Injections into the facet joints or blocks of the nerves that go to the facets can be very helpful in relieving back pain. As with all other injections, however, facet blocks should not be used in isolation, but rather in conjunction with a rehabilitation program stressing muscle flexibility, strengthening, and functional restoration.

Manipulation Under Joint Anesthesia

As the name implies, Manipulation Under Joint Anesthesia (MUJA) is a state-of-the-art procedure that combines two treatment modalities aimed at relieving pain coming from facet syndrome. MUJA is reserved for patients who have not responded to, or had only short term results with, traditional treatments for back pain (chiropractic, physical therapy, medications, etc.). It serves to address spinal joint pain (facet syndromes) that is both mechanical and inflammatory.

During the MUJA procedure, the patient lies on an exam table and undergoes a targeted injection of medications, including a local anesthetic to numb the region and a corticosteroid to reduce inflammation around the joint. After the injection, the patient is put through a series of passive (relaxed) stretches aimed at lengthening spinal muscles and soft tissues. This is followed by a specific manipulation procedure to the anesthetized spinal joints.

I have personally performed MUJA on hundreds of patients with very good results. Research thus far has concluded that MUJA may be a new, promising avenue in the treatment of chronic back pain. We are currently involved in a large-scale study on MUJA to show its effectiveness when compared to facet injections or manipulation alone.

Nerve Blocks

Another common injection, a selective nerve root block or simply "nerve block," is primarily used as a means to help diagnose the specific source of nerve pain and, secondarily, for therapeutic relief of low-back or leg pain. Nerve blocks are injections of anesthetics, steroids, and opioids onto or near nerves. In some cases of severe pain it is even necessary to destroy a nerve with injections of phenol, pure ethanol, or by using needles that freeze or heat the nerves.

When a nerve root becomes compressed and inflamed, it may produce back or leg pain. If imaging studies are unable to clearly show which nerve is causing the pain, a nerve block injection is performed to help determine which nerve is the source of pain. If your pain goes away after the injection, it can be inferred that the back pain was caused by the specific nerve root that has just been injected.

In addition to its diagnostic function, nerve blocks can be a very effective way to help manage pain, particularly for chronic pain sufferers. An injection of local anesthetic and steroid to the nerve root will block the nerve and reduce inflammation. This technique can also block one or two small nerves that convey pain messages to and from the facet joint and spinal cord. Success rates vary depending on the primary diagnosis and whether or not the injections are being used primarily for diagnosis or therapy.

Manipulation Post-Epidural Steroid Injection (MPESI)

This procedure is similar to MUJA but utilizes epidural steroid injections followed by manipulation as an attempt to address both mechanical and inflammatory pain emanating from spinal nerves.

Trigger Point Injections

Myofascial trigger points are "knots" in the muscle that when pressure is applied, cause pain in both the location of the trigger point and in other areas of the body. For example, putting pressure on a trigger point at the base of the neck will elicit pain in the forehead, and putting pressure on a trigger point in the middle of the low back may result in pain in your side. This unique trait of trigger points is called 'referred pain.'

Trigger points are difficult to properly diagnose in the acute stages of low back pain when muscle spasm and inflammation are present. Initially, trigger points generally respond to a program of stretching, deep tissue massage, and the correction of poor posture with other therapies such as superficial heat or cold. Trigger point injections are typically used in those who have not responded in the first four to six weeks of more conservative therapies.

Trigger points are often successfully treated with a course of local injections of a small dose of anesthetic such as lidocaine and are usually used as a part of a more comprehensive treatment program.

Manipulation Under Anesthesia (MUA)

Manipulation Under Anesthesia (MUA) is the use of manual manipulation of the spine combined with the use of general anesthetic. The addition of anesthetic allows for the benefits of manipulation to be shared with those patients who cannot tolerate manual techniques because of pain response, spasm, muscle contractures, and guarding.

Manipulation Under Anesthesia has been practiced since the late 1930's and has been used by chiropractors, osteopathic physicians, and orthopedic surgeons for many years as a proven form of treatment. It is a multi-disciplinary outpatient procedure that takes place in a controlled hospital or ambulatory surgical setting, usually over the course of one to three days. Using specialized chiropractic techniques supported by the expertise of M.D.s, R.N.s, and anesthesiologists, MUA achieves maximum results for qualified patients.

When combined with other forms of chiropractic care and rehabilitation, MUA procedures are very effective for a number of conditions; and, in many cases, are the treatment of choice over more invasive surgical procedures or steroid injections.

Performing MUA often involves hospital privileges and requires extensive post-graduate training. I personally have undergone extensive training and certification in M.U.A. for chronic pain cases.

Surgery

The rate of spinal surgery in the United States is 40% higher than in any other country. For this reason, except in severe cases, spinal surgery is reserved for patients who have failed with other, less invasive, treatments.

According to the March-June 2004 issue of *Disability Medicine*, surgery for degenerative disc disease is indicated only in cases of chronic (over 6-months) low back pain whose symptoms have failed with aggressive non-operative care.

The October 1988 issue of *The Archives of Physical Medicine & Rehabiltation* indicates that only 1-2% of back pain cases require surgery. The authors go on to state that pain alone is not a reason for surgery, and the only absolute reason to have surgery is loss of bowel or bladder control from a large disc herniation (known as cauda equina syndrome).

In a 1988 presentation to the North American Spine Society, Jeffrey Saal, M.D., and Joel Saal, M.D., concluded that "herniated nucleus pulposis with radiculopathy can be treated very successfully with non-operative care."

When all other therapies fail to relieve your pain, or if there is significant compression of the spine or nerves that can lead to permanent nerve damage, surgery may be the option of choice. As you read earlier, there are several conditions that may cause neural impingement including spinal stenosis, a disc herniation, spondylolisthesis, or a spinal tumor. There are two general types of lower back surgery that comprise the most common lumbar surgical procedures: decompression and spinal fusion.

Decompression is a surgical procedure that is performed to alleviate pain by removing sections of disc or bone that are putting pressure on a nerve (neural impingement). In this type of back surgery, a small portion of the bone over the nerve root and/or disc material from under the nerve root is removed to give the nerve root more space and provide a better healing environment.

There are two common types of spine surgery decompression procedures: a microdiscectomy – where a small piece of a disc is removed – or a laminectomy – where a small piece of the vertebral bone is removed. Sometimes in addition to the decompression procedure, a spinal fusion surgery is also necessary in order to achieve adequate decompression of a nerve root.

A spinal fusion surgery is designed to stop the motion at a painful vertebral segment, which in turn should decrease pain generated from the joint. All lumbar spinal fusion surgery involves adding bone graft to an area of the spine to set up a biological response that causes the bone graft to grow between the two vertebral elements and thereby stopping the motion at that segment.

In general, a lumbar spinal fusion surgery is most effective for those conditions involving only one vertebral segment. Most patients will not notice any limitation in motion after a one-level spinal fusion. However, spinal fusion of more than two segments is unlikely to provide pain relief because it removes too much of the normal motion in the lower back and places too much stress across the remaining joints. Only in rare cases should a three-level (or more) fusion surgery for pain alone be considered, although it may be necessary in cases of scoliosis, fracture, or deformity.

Only a minority of people with back problems need surgery. If your doctor suggests an operation, you will probably have already tried several other treatments unsuccessfully.

10

Prehab: Exercises to Prevent Pain

"A man's health can be judged by which he takes two at a time - pills or stairs."

- Joan Welsh

The Foundations of Spinal Health

As we have discussed in the previous sections of this book, the human body is an amazingly complex system of bones, joints, muscles, and nerves, designed to work together to accomplish one thing: movement. Everything about the human body is designed with movement in mind – nerve fibers stimulate the muscles to contract, muscles contract to move the bones, bones move around joints, and the nervous system controls it all.

As a matter of fact, research has shown that movement is so critical to our body's health that a lack of movement has a detrimental affect on everything from digestion to our emotional state, immune function, our ability to concentrate, how well we sleep, and even how long we live. The bottom line is that if your lifestyle does not include enough movement, your body cannot function efficiently. Consequently, three things will happen. First, you will not be as physically healthy and will suffer from a wide variety of physical ailments, ranging from headaches to high blood pressure. Second, you will not be as productive in your life because of reduced energy levels and the ability to mentally focus. Third, because you have less energy, your activity level will tend to drop off even further over time, creating a downward spiral of reduced energy and less activity until you get to a point where even the demands of a sedentary job leave you physically exhausted by the end of the day.

Foundation One: Posture

The most immediate problem with poor posture is that it creates chronic muscle tension as the weight of the head and upper body is having to be supported by the muscles instead of the bones. This effect becomes more pronounced the further your posture deviates from your center of gravity.

To illustrate this idea further, think about carrying a briefcase. If you had to carry a briefcase with your arms outstretched in front of you, it would not take long before the muscles of your shoulders would be completely exhausted. This is because carrying the briefcase far away from your center of gravity places undue stress on your shoulder muscles. If you held the same briefcase down at your side, your muscles would not fatigue as quickly because the briefcase is closer to your center of gravity and the weight is, therefore, supported by the bones of the skeleton, rather than the muscles.

Correcting bad posture and the physical problems that result are accomplished by doing two things. The first is to eliminate as much 'bad' stress from your body as possible. Bad stress includes all the factors, habits, or stressors that cause

Your Center of Gravity

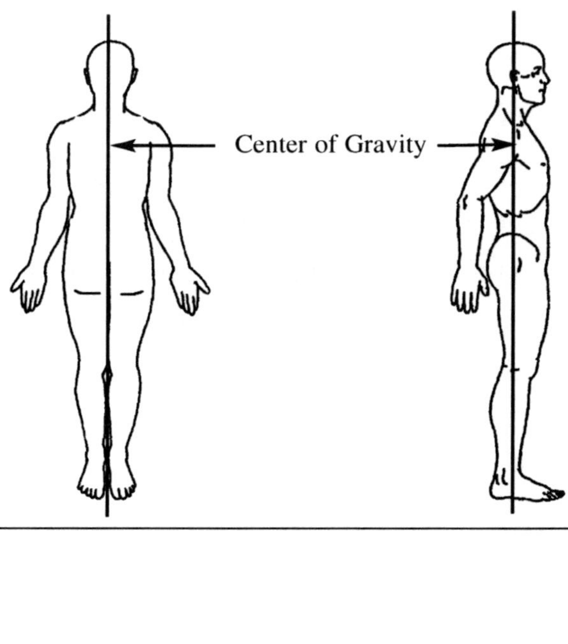

your body to deviate from your center of gravity. This can include having a poorly adjusted workstation, not having your seat adjusted correctly in your car, or even carrying too much weight around in a heavy purse or backpack.

The second is to apply 'good' stress on the body in an effort to move your posture back toward your center of gravity. Getting your body back to its center of gravity by improving your posture is critically important to improving how you feel. This is accomplished through a series of exercises, stretches, adjustments, and changes to your physical environment that all work to help correct your posture.

Foundation Two: Movement

Imagine waking up one morning with a frozen shoulder where you couldn't move your upper arm more than a few inches in any direction. How much would that impact your ability to do your job? How much would that affect your ability to drive your car or even to dress yourself? How much would that affect your ability to concentrate on anything other than your shoulder? Obviously, if your shoulder did not move correctly, it would have a dramatic impact on your life. The same is true with movement in every part of your body. If things aren't moving the way they are supposed to move, it will have a negative impact on your ability to function at work and take care of the demands of everyday life, including your ability to concentrate.

Over the years, I have had a number of patients come into my office with severe low back pain who stated that their pain came on suddenly when they did something as simple as bend down to pet their cat, put on their socks, or pick up the newspaper. Just about everyone would agree that a person's body should be able to handle something as simple as bending over to pick up a newspaper or putting on their socks, right? So what happened?

In every one of these cases, I have found that many of the joints in their body were barely moving at all; they were hypomobile or locked up. When the joints in one area of the body do not move the way they should, other areas of the body are forced to move more than they were designed to in an effort to compensate for the area that is not moving. This creates significant stress on the areas that are having to pick up the slack of the joints that aren't moving properly. This can lead to pain and inflammation. At the same time, those joints without normal movement can continue to stick together, causing the ligaments and tendons to shorten. This leaves the body in an unstable condition, and if left unchecked, can progress until the body can hardly move at all. This will cause the person to suffer flare-ups of pain at even the slightest provocation.

Most of us have seen people who have lost most of their normal mobility. This is especially prevalent among the elderly. Contrary to popular belief, this is not the inevitable effect of aging, rather it is the unfortunate effect of not maintaining the body's mobility through exercise, stretching, healthy alignment, and body mechanics. There are a lot of people in their 60s, 70s, or even older, who are stronger and more flexible than the average person in their 30s simply because they keep themselves strong and flexible through exercise. Maintaining mobility is critical in order to live free from pain and disability. Maintaining good mobility is not difficult, but it does not happen on its own.

Just as in developing a good posture, it is necessary that you perform specific exercises and stretches to keep your muscles, ligaments, and tendons flexible and healthy. In addition, it is crucial that all of the joints in your body move properly. Although this can be achieved to a great degree through the stretches described in this book, most people also find routine chiropractic adjustments to be very beneficial.

Foundation Three: Strength

Strong muscles keep your body upright and allow you to move. Good muscle strength and balance are critical for proper posture and to minimize muscle tension. Your muscles function much like the wires that hold up a tall radio or television antenna. If the wires are equally strong on all sides, the antenna will stand up straight. If one of the wires becomes weak or breaks, the antenna will either lean to the side or collapse. The same is true with your body. If the muscles on all sides of your spine are balanced and strong, your body will stand up straight and strong. Unfortunately, most people don't have balanced and strong muscles. The reason for this gets back to lack of exercise and abnormal motion of the spine.

Muscles are very efficient at getting stronger or weaker in response to the demands placed on them. Since most of us sit at a desk, drive a car, and sit on the sofa at home, many of our muscles are not challenged. Consequently, they become weak. At the same time, the muscles that are constantly used throughout the day become strong. This imbalance of muscle strength contributes to poor posture and chronic muscle tension. Left unchecked, muscle imbalances tend to get worse, not better, because of a phenomenon called "Reciprocal Inhibition."

Reciprocal Inhibition literally means "shutting down the opposite." Simply put, for all of the muscles that move your body in one direction, there are opposing muscles that move the body in the opposite direction. In order to keep these muscles from working against each other, when the body contracts one muscle group, it forces the opposing group to relax – it shuts down the opposite muscles.

This phenomenon is especially important to people who work at a desk because all day long the same muscles in the upper back and chest area of the body are used. This means that throughout the day, the body is essentially shutting down the opposite muscles in the middle back. Over time, the muscles in the middle back become very weak because they are not being worked like the muscles in the front. This contributes to poor posture and chronic muscle spasm and pain.

Reciprocal Inhibition

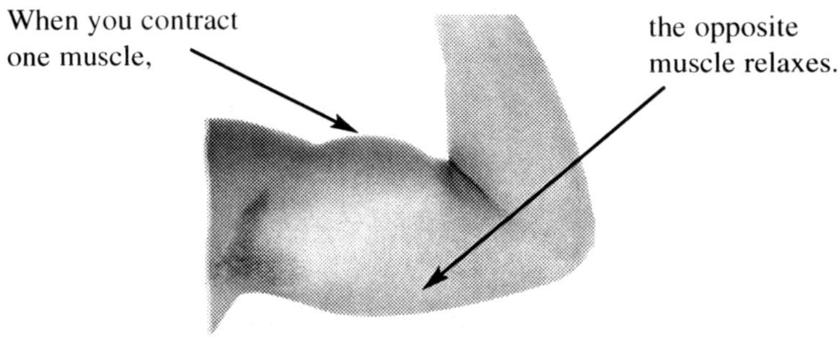

Reciprocal Inhibition keeps opposing muscle groups from working against each other and allows the body to move with smooth and effortless motion.

The easiest way to correct this imbalance is to learn and perform specific exercises which will increase the strength of the back muscles, along with manual therapy and chiropractic care. Once the muscles in your middle back are strong, the resultant tightness and poor posture often disappear.

Foundation Four: Coordination

Healthy coordination is the result of using the body in the manner in which it was designed. Exercises such as walking, swimming, rock climbing, yoga, pilates, bicycling, martial arts, and body building all help to improve muscle coordination, whereas working at a desk, reading, and watching television do the opposite. Without realizing it, most people are in a dramatic state of muscle imbalance. This occurs simply because they sit for many hours every day and do not perform exercises on a regular basis that will work to keep all of the muscles in their body properly coordinated. This muscular imbalance contributes to muscle tightness, restricted movement, and joint pain.

The Importance of Exercise

Everyone knows that exercise is important for good health. Study after study has shown that exercise is effective at decreasing pain, reducing stress, improving immune function, lowering blood pressure, improving cardiac function, boosting energy, improving sleep, and maintaining a healthy body weight. The fact remains that although most people are aware of how important exercise is to their health, they still do not exercise the way that they should.

In their landmark book entitled Biomarkers, medical researchers, Dr. William Evans and Dr. Irwin Rosenberg identified several characteristic changes that occur as we age including a loss of muscle mass, a decrease in strength, a decrease in basal metabolic rate, a decrease in aerobic capacity, an increase in blood pressure, a loss of normal insulin action, a decrease in circulating HDL to total cholesterol ratio, a loss of bone density, and a decreased ability to control your body temperature. Each one of these measures of physical health tends to decline as we age. What Evans and Rosenberg discovered is that exercise was effective in reversing every single one of these markers of aging!

You don't have to exercise as intensely as Lance Armstrong or Arnold Schwarzenegger to enjoy the benefits of exercise. But you do have to get up and get your body moving at least five or six days per week, preferably doing a combination of aerobic exercise and strength training. This will help you not only feel better and have more energy, but will help to stabilize and strengthen your whole body.

Types of Exercise

As a former personal trainer, I am a huge proponent of regular exercise. Research has shown that certain exercises may reduce your chance of back or neck pain. My patients are given a specific regimen of exercises while under my care, and the protocol is tailored towards their specific condition.

In this chapter, I will introduce you to basic exercise concepts. I will also show you several muscle stretches and exercises that, when performed regularly, can help you prevent muscular imbalances, weakness, and incoordination that may lead to future spinal problems.

Aerobic Exercise

Aerobic means "using oxygen" and aerobic exercises are those that utilize oxygen during the activity. Aerobic exercise trains the body to utilize oxygen more efficiently and improves your overall cardiovascular fitness. Aerobic activities are those that are performed for an extended period of time at a low intensity. Examples of aerobic activities are biking, aerobic walking, swimming, jogging, in-line skating, aerobic dance, cross-country skiing, and using an elliptical trainer. The benefits of aerobic activity include

- Improved breathing.
- Increased energy throughout the day.
- Improved heart health and cardiac output.
- Decreased blood pressure.
- Decreased serum cholesterol.
- Decreased stress.
- More restful sleep.
- Improved mood and mental functioning.
- Improved digestion and bowel function.

For maximum benefit, you should engage in at least 20 minutes of aerobic activity five or six days per week. If you already do more than this, great! For those who have not engaged in regular activity for a while, even 20 minutes a day will be a significant accomplishment.

During aerobic exercise, you should be able to carry on a conversation without feeling too winded. If you are breathing too heavy to carry on a conversation easily, you should ease up a bit. As you become healthier, you will be able to increase the intensity of your activity without feeling short of breath.

This brings up another important point - a concept called the overload principle. The overload principle simply states that in order to benefit from physical activity, the intensity has to be greater than what your body is used to. Only by pushing your body a little bit - by overloading it - will your body respond by growing stronger.

Strength Training

Strength training differs from aerobic training in three important ways. First, strength training involves activities that are more intense and much shorter in duration than aerobic activity, for example doing push-ups or sit-ups. Second, while aerobic training primarily improves the health of your cardiovascular system, strength training primarily improves the health of your muscles, bones, and joints. Third, while aerobic activity should be performed almost every day for maximum benefit, you only need to engage in strength training two to three times per week in order to maximize the effects of training. The benefits of strength training include the following:

- increased muscle and bone strength
- improved muscle tone and body shape
- improved hormone function
- improved mood and mental functioning
- decreased serum cholesterol

- decreased stress
- more restful sleep
- increased metabolism

To benefit from strength training, it is not necessary that you spend long grueling hours in the gym every day. In fact, you can experience a significant improvement in your strength and muscle tone by weightlifting for one hour, just two or three times a week!

The key to successful strength training is not the amount of time you spend; it is the intensity that is important. The harder you work your muscles during your strength workouts, the quicker you will see improvements. Each time you exercise your muscles hard, your body goes to work to build more muscle. As long as you continue to slowly increase the weight that you use week after week, your muscles will continue to grow in strength. Most people begin to see a difference in their strength and how they look after a few weeks of strength training.

Stretching

Stretching not only feels great; it is also very effective at reducing muscle tension, decreasing stress, and maintaining flexibility and joint mobility. In order to experience the benefits of stretching, however, it is important that you stretch correctly. Stretching your muscles too hard, bouncing while holding a stretch, or stretching your muscles when they are too cold can injure your muscles and lead to muscle tightness. Proper stretching technique is easy provided you follow a few simple rules.

The first rule is to never stretch your muscles too hard. You should only stretch to the point where you feel a mild pull on the muscle. If you attempt to stretch further, you may cause small muscle tears and create a reflex tightening of the muscle. Repetitive overstretching can cause scarring of the muscle and a loss of flexibility.

The second rule is to never bounce while stretching. When you bounce, you momentarily force your muscles to overstretch and increase your risk of muscular injury.

The third rule is to only stretch your muscles when they are warm. Muscles are a lot like plastic. If you heat plastic, you can bend it and stretch it without breaking. By stretching once you are warmed up, stretching will be much more safe and effective.

The Magnificent Seven: Exercises to Prevent Back and Neck Pain

The following exercises should be done at least every other day. They should be performed in the exact order shown, as I have designed the program to both strengthen and stretch the key spinal muscles.

When starting this or any exercise program, please note the following:

Always check with your doctor before starting any exercise program. Stop the exercise if you experience any discomfort or pain. Remember, these stretches and exercises are meant to create flexibility and strength, so minor discomfort from these movements is normal. Ease into this program. Start slow, and add repetitions or sets as you progress.

1. Lay on your back, with your knees bent and feet flat on the floor. Slowly rotate your pelvis, flattening your spine against the floor. As you do this, gently "hollow" your stomach, feeling your belly button press against your spine, while at the same time tightening your buttock muscles. Hold this position for 3 seconds and repeat 10 times.

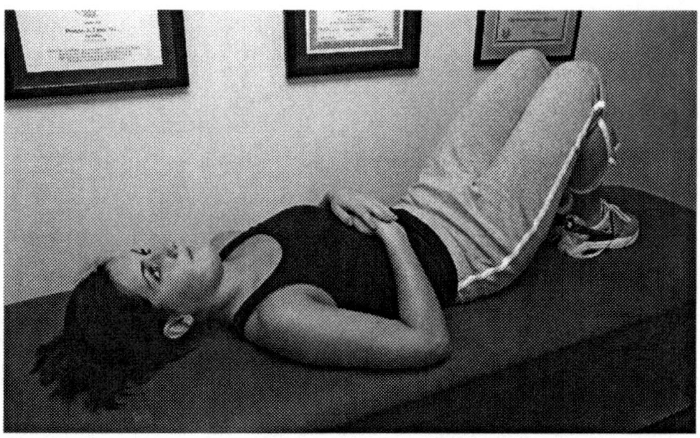

2. While still on your back, keep your spine straight (not arched), and tighten your stomach muscles while pushing down on your heels and slowly raising your buttocks off the floor. Hold this position for three seconds and repeat 10 times.

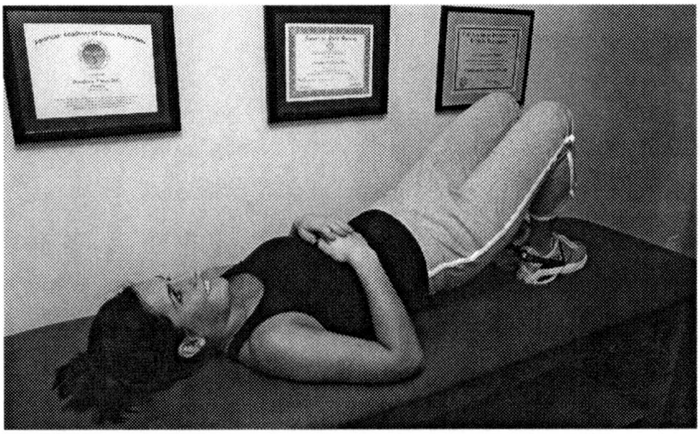

3. Now, roll over to a comfortable position on the floor with your hands directly below your shoulders and your knees directly under your hips.

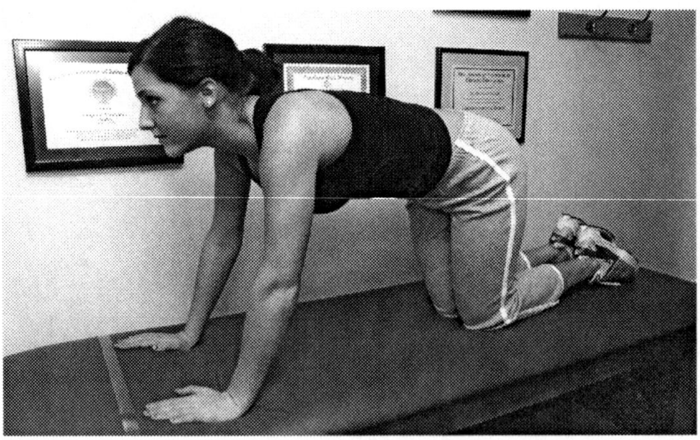

4. Slowly tuck your chin and tighten your stomach muscles as you arch your back. Hold for a count of 3.

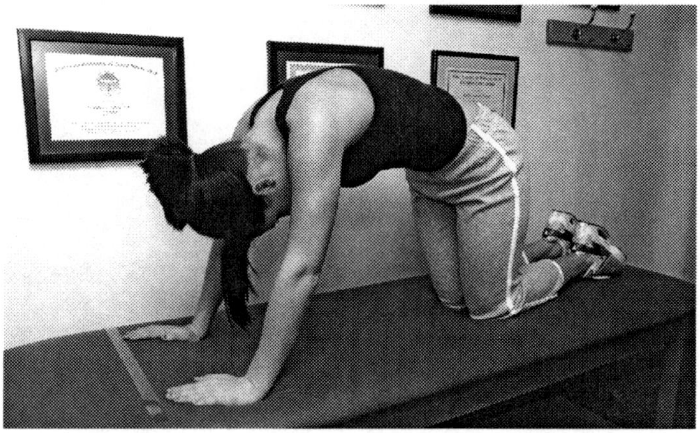

Then slowly allow your stomach muscles to relax and let your mid-back sag. Repeat this cycle, arching and sagging, for a total of 10 repetitions.

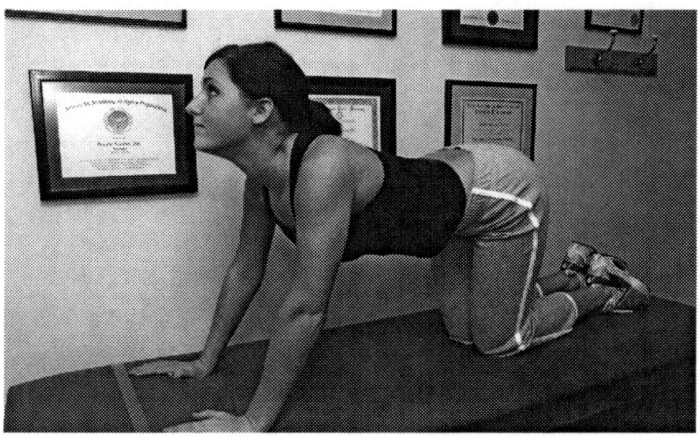

5. Assume a neutral spine position.

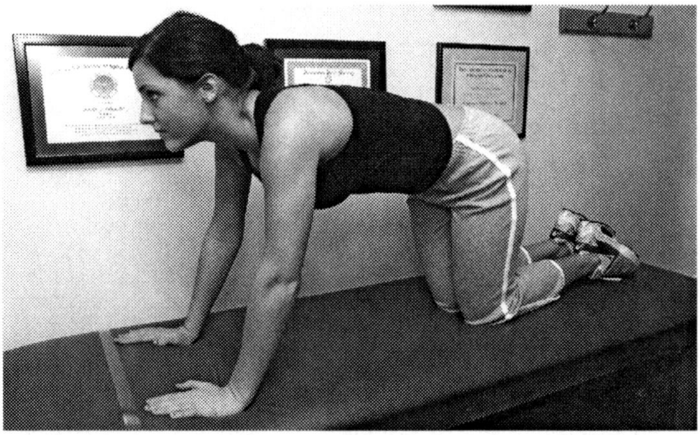

While keeping your neck and back straight and stable, raise one arm out forward in front of you. Hold for a count of three, then lower the arm and repeat with the opposite arm. Alternate each arm 15 times.

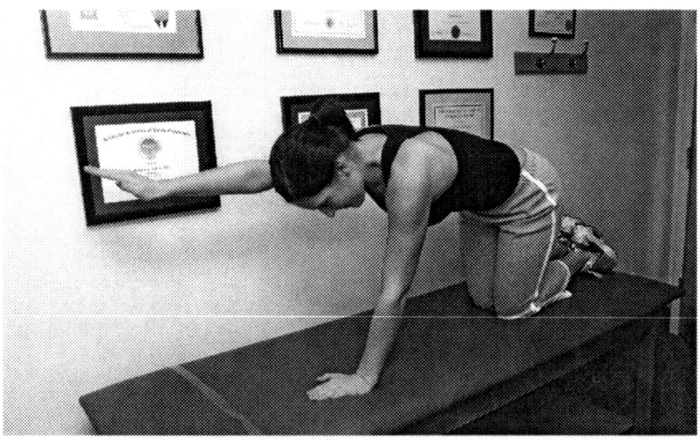

6. Then, while still keeping your neck and back straight and stable, raise one leg behind you. Be careful not to elevate the leg past the point where it is even with your low back. Repeat this with the opposite leg, and alternate for a total of 10 repetitions for each leg.

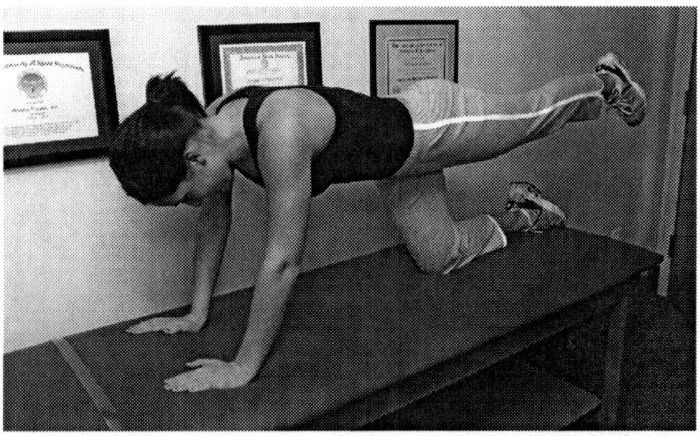

7. Return to neutral, and while continuing to keep your spine straight and stable, slowly raise the opposite arm and leg for a total of 15 sets of each.

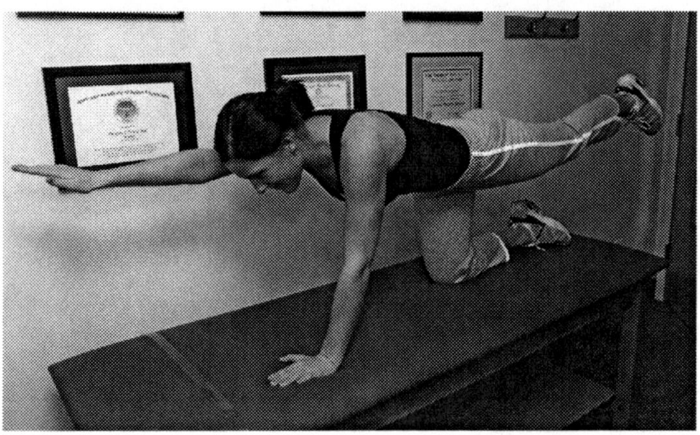

The Triple Threat: Daily Neck Exercises

These daily exercises can be easily performed at home or your workplace, and are often useful as a "stress break."

1. Sitting comfortably, grasp your chair or reach behind your back with your left hand, while with your right hand gently (no bouncing) tilt your head to the right. Hold the stretch for 3 seconds. Repeat this 5 times on the right, and then switch to the left. Repeat the exercise.

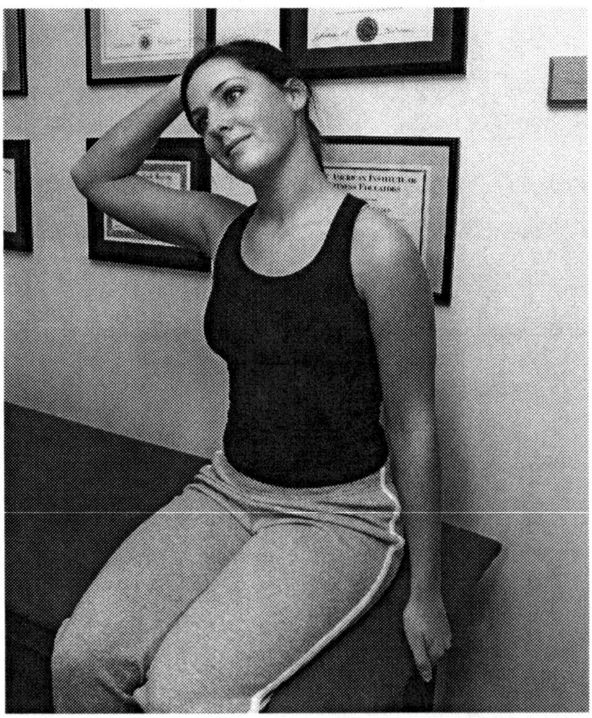

2. Rest your left hand on your left shoulder blade as shown. Turn your head to the right, and, using your right hand gently pull your head in a diagonal direction until a gentle stretch is felt. Hold for 3 seconds. Repeat the stretch on the opposite side. Perform a total of 5 stretches per side.

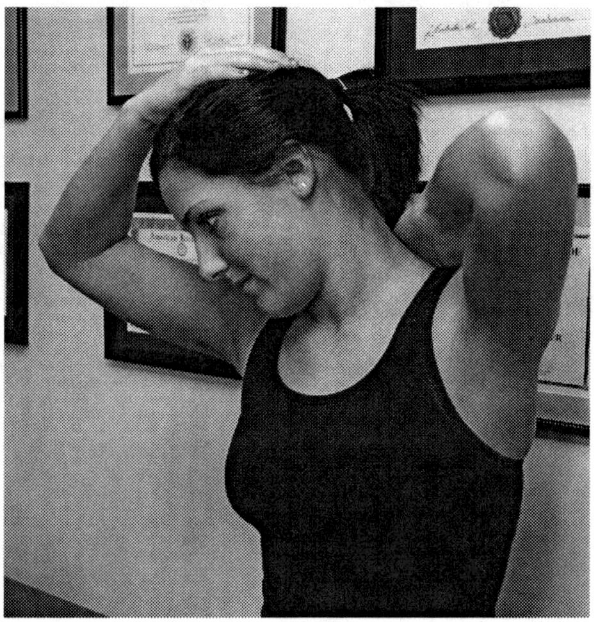

3. Stand in an open doorway and place your hands at shoulder level on the door frame. Slowly (no bouncing!) lean forward until you feel a gentle stretch across the chest and front shoulders. Hold for 3 seconds and repeat 5 times.

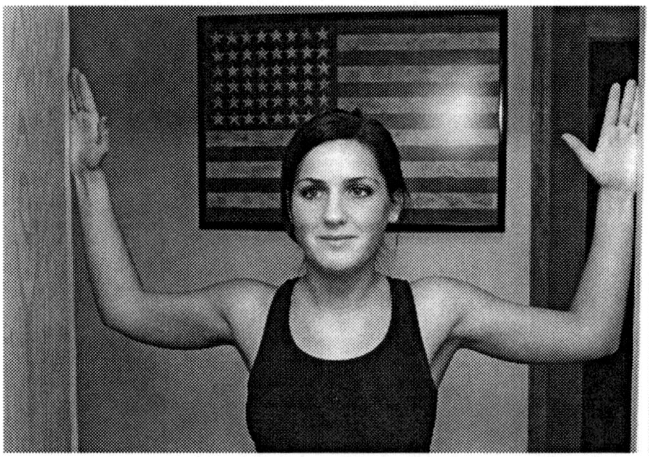

11

Nutrition

"Each patient carries his own doctor inside him. They come to us not knowing that truth. We are at our best when we give the doctor who resides in each patient a chance to work."

- Albert Schweitzer, M.D.

Food is not simply an energy source for the body. Each piece of food you put into your mouth contains hundreds or thousands of individual chemicals that influence a wide range of functions in your body including your metabolic rate, immune function, emotional state, and even your body weight. It is important to understand how carbohydrates, proteins, and fats influence your body's biochemistry so that you can make informed choices about the foods you eat. Once you understand some simple ideas about food, you can use this knowledge to improve your overall health. In this chapter, you will learn how your body uses the three basic types of food - carbohydrates, fats, and proteins. You will also learn about certain vitamins, minerals, and herbs that are critical to your overall health.

Carbohydrates

Carbohydrates are the main fuel source that your body uses to think, run, walk, breathe, and perform just about every action. Next to water, carbohydrates are the most consumed nutrients in the world. There are three types of carbohydrates that you consume every day: sugars, complex carbohydrates, and fiber.

In order for the body to use the sugars and starches in food, it must first break them down to a form that can be used by your body's cells. The first step of the digestion processes occurs in your mouth by an enzyme called salivary amylase. This enzyme begins the process of breaking down starches into simple sugars. Once the food reaches your stomach, the digestion of carbohydrates stops. It begins again once your food leaves the stomach and enters the small intestine.

The main purpose of the digestion process is to convert the carbohydrate you consumed into a simple sugar called glucose. Glucose is the primary fuel source for the brain, central nervous system, and nearly every other cell in your body.

To ensure a readily available supply of glucose, the body stores it in the muscle and liver in a form called glycogen. Glycogen is then converted back to glucose any time your blood glucose level drops too low. If your body uses up all its glycogen, it will start breaking down muscle in order to provide your vital organs with the glucose they need to function.

The two major hormones that help regulate the level of glucose in your blood are insulin and glucagon. Insulin is a hormone that is released when your blood glucose levels rise, as typically occurs after you consume food containing carbohydrates. The function of insulin is to signal the liver and muscle cells to remove the excess glucose from the blood and store it as glycogen.

Glucagon has the opposite effect. When your blood glucose levels become too low, glucagon will signal the muscle

Blood Glucose, Insulin, and Glucagon

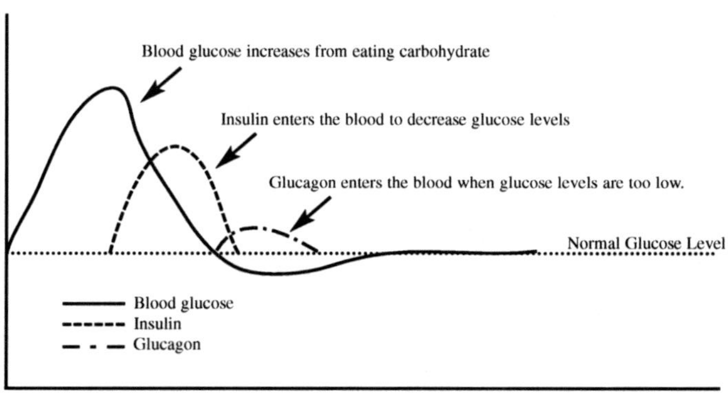

and liver to convert glycogen back to glucose and release it into the blood stream. The balance of these two hormones helps to keep blood glucose levels within a fairly narrow range.

There are some instances where the body is unable to maintain healthy blood glucose levels. The most common condition is called diabetes and is caused by a loss of normal insulin function. Those with diabetes have an abnormally high blood glucose level. A much rarer condition called primary hypoglycemia is when blood glucose levels are abnormally low.

Not all carbohydrates have the same effect on blood glucose levels. Starches are much larger molecules than sugars and therefore take longer to break down and enter the blood stream as glucose. Sugars, on the other hand, are simple molecules that can quickly be converted into glucose and enter the blood. Sugars will tend to create a sharp spike in blood glucose levels, whereas starches will tend to cause a much more gradual increase.

The measure of a food's ability to elevate blood glucose levels is referred to as its glycemic index. Simple sugars have a high glycemic index because they cause a very rapid increase in blood glucose levels. Larger, more complex carbohydrates such as starches have a low glycemic index because they cause a gradual increase in blood glucose levels.

High glycemic index foods - foods that contain a lot of sugar - will tend to increase your storage of body fat. The reason is that each fat cell in your body can also respond to

Glycemic Index and Insulin Resistance

A high glycemic index (GI) carbohydrate is one that causes a very rapid and substantial increase in blood sugar. Foods such as ice cream, cake, sugared breakfast cereals, and candy bars fall into the category of high glycemic index foods. Surprisingly, so do many foods that are commonly considered healthy, such as bananas, orange juice, pineapple, and watermelon.

Low glycemic index foods are those that have a much lower and slower effect on your body's blood glucose levels. This includes high protein foods, such as meat and eggs, as well as beans, legumes, most vegetables, and high-fiber whole grain foods.

When your diet consists of a lot of high glycemic index foods, your body will secrete an excess amount of insulin in an effort to keep your blood sugar levels down. This causes much of the carbohydrate you consume to be stored directly into your fat cells, leading to an increase in body fat.

The other serious detrimental effect of these spikes in blood sugar and insulin has to do with the fact that when your insulin levels peak at high levels several times per day, your muscles and liver, which are important for storing blood glucose, stop reacting to the insulin's message to store some of the sugar that is floating around in the blood. This phenomenon is called insulin resistance.

When insulin resistance develops, your body produces insulin in response to your blood sugar rising, but your body no longer uses the insulin properly, causing your blood sugar levels to remain high. Insulin resistance not only contributes to being overweight, but it is also is the precursor for a serious condition called Type II, or adult-onset, diabetes.

The four most effective ways to combat insulin resistance are to consume only low glycemic index foods, eat smaller meals more frequently throughout the day, supplement with chromium and alpha-lipoic acid, and perform some type of aerobic exercise each day.

insulin, take glucose out of the blood, and store it. But instead of storing the extra glucose as glycogen like the muscles and liver do, it stores the excess glucose as fat. The higher your blood glucose rises, the more of it will be stored in your fat cells. To minimize the amount of carbohydrate that ends up being stored as fat, it is important that you consume low glycemic index foods such as whole grains and pastas.

Carbohydrates are an essential part of any healthy diet, especially when you are on a weight loss program. It is important to stick to the low glycemic index carbs to avoid elevating your blood glucose to the point where the carbs end up being stored as fat.

Proteins

Proteins are required to maintain the normal structure and function of the body. Whereas carbohydrates, especially glucose, are the primary fuel source for the body, proteins are used as the primary building blocks of the body tissues such as muscle, bone, and connective tissue. In addition, the enzymes, antibodies, hemoglobin, and even your DNA are all made from protein.

Proteins are made up of about 20 different amino acids. Twelve of these amino acids can be synthesized in your body and, therefore, do not need to come from your diet. These are called the non-essential amino acids. The other eight amino acids are essential amino acids and need to come from your diet including isoleucine, leucine, lysine, methionine, phenylalanine, threonine, tryptophan and valine. If you do not get enough of these amino acids in your diet, your body cannot repair itself, your immune system can't do its job properly, your metabolism will decrease, and you will tend to feel sluggish, depressed, and tired. The primary sources of these amino acids are from protein sources such as meat, fish, cheese, eggs, soy, dairy products, beans, and legumes.

Before your body can use the protein in your food, it must first break down the protein to its individual amino acids. Digestion of protein begins in the stomach where acids and proteolytic enzymes begin the process of releasing amino acids from the protein. Some amino acids are absorbed directly through the stomach lining and enter into the blood stream. The remaining protein then enters the small intestine where digestion is completed.

Once the amino acids enter the blood, the body can use them to build red blood cells, muscle tissue, immune factors, or whatever else the body needs. However, all twenty amino acids must be present in the blood in the proper ratios in order for the body to manufacture new proteins. If one amino acid is missing or is present in a very limited quantity, then that amino acid becomes the limiting factor to protein synthesis. For this reason, it is best to eat proteins that have all of the amino acids that the body needs.

The proteins in some foods have amino acid profiles that very closely match the ratios that the human body needs such

Biological Value of Proteins

Protein Source	BV*	PD**	
Whey Protein Concentrate		104	99%
Whole Egg		100	98%
Cow's Milk		91	
Egg White	88		
Fish		83	
Beef		80	98%
Chicken		79	
Casein		77	99%
Rice		74	
Soy		74	95%
Wheat		54	91%
Beans		49	
Peanuts		43	

* Biological Value - how well the amino acid profile of the food matches the needs of the body.
** Percentage of Digestion - how well the protein is digested and absorbed in the body.

as eggs, dairy, and meat. These proteins are said to have a high biological value (BV). Eggs are considered to have the highest biological value and are used as the standard by which all other proteins are compared. In the Biological Value of Proteins chart, you will see that eggs have a BV score of 100. The 100 represents that approximately 100% of the protein in eggs can be metabolized by the body because it so closely matches the amino acid profile of the body.

Other foods such as grains, vegetables, and beans have amino acid profiles that do not match the body's needs very well. These are lower biological quality proteins and have lower BV scores.

You will notice that whey (milk) protein concentrate has a BV of 104. Is it possible to have a 104% of the milk proteins absorbed? Well, no. When the standard of biological value was initially set, egg protein had the best amino acid profile of any protein known at the time, so eggs were made the standard and given a value of 100. Since then, it was discovered that highly concentrated whey protein from milk actually had a slightly better amino acid profile than eggs. Instead of changing the standard to whey, it was decided to just give whey protein a score of more than 100.

The other measure of the overall quality of protein is how much of the protein can be digested by your body - the Percentage of Digestion (PD) score. Some proteins such as bone, cartilage, and tendon may have a high biological value because of their amino acid profiles but are completely non-digestible and, therefore, your body can't absorb the amino acids they contain. When you are cutting back on your overall food intake in an effort to lose weight, it is important to eat higher biological value proteins as well as those with the highest digestibility (PD).

Proteins have an added advantage in that they don't cause a rapid increase in blood glucose levels, which makes them low glycemic index foods. In addition, proteins will increase your body's metabolism more than carbohydrates and fats and will provide the building blocks for many mood-elevating neuro-transmitters such as serotonin and dopamine.

Proteins are critical for building lean muscle tissue, maintaining stable blood glucose levels, immune function, and normal brain chemistry. Since proteins that have a higher biological value are those that have an amino acid profile that closely match the needs for the body, eating higher biological value proteins have the advantage of giving you the greatest amount of usable protein for the number of calories consumed.

Fats

Of the three major components of food, fats are certainly the most misunderstood and the most villainized. Fat is not the bad thing that it is often made out to be. Your brain, spinal cord, and entire nervous system are largely made from fat as well as many of your hormones such as testosterone and estrogen. Fat provides your body with a store of energy and insulation from the cold, and it protects your organs from physical damage. In fact, next to water, fat is the most abundant substance in the human body, ideally averaging about 10% - 20% of a person's total body weight.

Dietary fats are necessary for the proper absorption of fat-soluble vitamins, and scientists have recently discovered that some fats in the diet are used for sending signals to the brain to control how much you eat. It is not fats, per se, that you should avoid. You should only avoid eating too much of the wrong kind of fat: saturated fat.

Dietary fats come in several forms: saturated fats, polyunsaturated fats, monounsaturated fats, and cholesterol. Saturated fats are the demons of dietary fats because they can elevate blood cholesterol which can lead to the development of heart disease. Saturated fats also tend to cause a low-grade inflammation in the body. Animal fats are the most common source of saturated fat in the diet. Other sources are snack foods, which usually contain a lot of palm oil and palm kernel oil. You will want to avoid saturated fats whenever possible by selecting lower-fat meats such as chicken, turkey, and pork and avoiding commercially prepared snack foods.

Polyunsaturated fats such as corn oil, flaxseed oil, or fish oils are much healthier forms of fat than saturated fats and tend to be liquid at room temperature, whereas saturated fats are usually solid. Unlike saturated fats, the polyunsaturates will help to decrease serum cholesterol, both LDL and HDL, and will help to decrease inflammation in the body.

Healthy and Unhealthy Fats

Saturated Fats - Unhealthy

Beef	Butter	Lard
Palm Oil	Palm Kernel Oil	Cheese
Whole Milk	Cocoa Butter	

Polyunsaturated Fats - Fairly Healthy

Corn Oil	Cottonseed Oil	Fish Oils
Safflower Oil	Soybean Oil	
Sunflower Oil	Mayonnaise	
Sesame Oil	Flaxseed Oil	

Monounsaturated Fats - Very Healthy

Canola Oil	Olive Oil	Avocados
Peanut Oil	Sesame Oil	Nuts

Monounsaturated fats are even healthier for your body than either saturated fats or polyunsaturated fats. They not only decrease your bad LDL cholesterol, but they also help raise your good HDL cholesterol! Using olive oil, canola oil, avocados, and nuts in the preparation of your daily meals is the simplest way to introduce monounsaturates into your diet.

Cholesterol is a waxy fat that is found exclusively in animal foods - beef, chicken, fish, turkey, eggs, dairy, etc. Years ago it was believed that consuming cholesterol in your diet led to an increase in your blood cholesterol, but this turned out to not be the case. Dietary cholesterol has very little, if any, impact on the blood cholesterol level of most people. The major contributors of cholesterol are eating too much saturated fat, being overweight, and not getting enough exercise.

Calories

A calorie is a measure of the energy content of food. Calories are what your body uses to keep your heart pumping, keep your lungs breathing, allow your mind to think, and give your muscles the energy they need. Carbohydrates and protein each provide four calories per gram, fats provide nine calories per gram, and alcohol provides approximately seven calories per gram. In other words, ounce for ounce, proteins and carbohydrates give you fewer than half of the calories of fat. The high caloric value of fat is why high-fat foods such as cream cheese and fried foods are so high in calories. It is important to

Calories of Common Foods

Food	CHO (g)	PRO (g)	FAT (g)	CAL
Meat / Eggs				
Beef, extra lean ground (3 oz.)	0	21	14	213
Chicken breast (3 oz.)	0	24	2	116
Eggs, cooked (2 eggs)	2	12	14	186
Ham, baked (3 oz.)	0	18	7	142
Lamb, baked (3 oz.)				
Pork tenderloin (3 oz.)	0	26	5	159
Tuna, in water (3 oz.)	0	22	0	99
Turkey breast (3 oz.)	0	20	1	100
Grains / Pasta				
Barley, cooked (1 cup)	44	4	1	193
Bread, 7-grain (1 slice)	17	4	2	100
Couscous, cooked (1 cup)	36	6	0	176
Oatmeal, cooked (1 cup)	28	6	1	134
Pasta, cooked (1 cup)	41	8	1	210
Potato, baked (1 medium)	51	5	0	220
Rice, brown, cooked (1 cup)	45	5	2	216
Vegetables				
Broccoli, fresh (1 cup)	4	2	0	20
Carrots, fresh (1 cup)	12	2	2	60
Cauliflower, fresh (1 cup)	5	2	0	25
Celery, fresh (1 cup)	4	1	0	19
Green beans, fresh (1 cup)	8	2	0	34
Green pepper, fresh (1 cup)	6	1	0	25
Peas, fresh (1 cup)	21	8	1	117
Fruits				
Apple (1 med.)	21	0	0	81
Banana (1 med.)	28	1	1	109
Orange (1 med.)	15	1	0	62
Pineapple (1 cup)	19	1	1	76
Raspberries (1 cup)	14	1	1	60

CHO = Carbohydrate (g) • PRO = Protein (g) • FAT = Fat (g) • CAL = Calories remember that calories are not your enemy. As strange as it may seem, if you don't eat enough food, it will be harder for you to lose weight because too much calorie restriction slows down your metabolism.

Maintaining a healthy body composition is a balancing act between the calories you consume and the calories you burn. We have spent some time discussing the main sources of energy in your diet - carbohydrates, proteins, and fats. Let's take a quick look at the other side of the equation - how your body burns the calories you consume.

Your body burns calories in two ways: your basal energy expenditure (also known as your basal metabolic rate) and your activity level. The biggest user of calories is your basal energy expenditure (BEE), which is the energy used by your organs to keep your body alive and to build muscles, bone, and connective tissue. Your BEE is responsible for burning up to three-fourths of all the calories you burn in one day.

Activity is the other way in which you burn calories. Depending on how active you are, activity can make up as little as fifteen percent or as much as thirty-five percent of the total calories you burn in a day.

Nutritional Supplements

I was recently told by a colleague that during a graduate nutrition course at the University of Minnesota, the professor posed a challenge to the class: Construct a 2000 calorie-per-day diet that at least met the Recommended Dietary Allowances (RDA) for vitamins and minerals without the use of supplements. After all, we have always heard that if you eat a well-balanced diet, you don't need to take vitamin supplements, right? Well, this professor was putting that statement to the test.

To everyone's surprise, no one was able to come up with a sustainable daily diet that met the minimum requirements for vitamin and mineral intake. The problem was not with getting the minimum vitamin intake; the challenge was getting enough of a few very important minerals, especially zinc. Unless you eat oysters or dark turkey meat every day, it is impossible to get the minimum RDA of zinc through diet alone.

The bottom line is that in order to get enough trace minerals in our diet to at least meet the minimum RDAs, it is necessary to take a good quality supplement.

Another argument for taking multivitamin and mineral supplements is that there is substantial evidence that taking doses of a class of nutrients called antioxidants, which far exceed the RDA minimums, can help prevent heart disease, help to mitigate some of the detrimental effects of diabetes, and help to promote healthy immune function.

In today's environment, you will be hard pressed to find a health care provider who does not recommend a multivitamin. I have designed a label called Once Daily Multi Vitamin which I recommend for patients who are not covering their dietary bases or who are taking a low quality, poorly absorbed multivitamin.

How To Choose a Supplement

All vitamin supplements are not created equal. Supplements are just like anything else - there are some good ones out there and a great deal of supplements that are not as good. Here a few ways to determine whether a particular vitamin is good:

- *In general, supplements sold through health care professionals are top quality. They tend to be a little more expensive than the supplements you find at your local drug store because the ingredients that go into them tend to be of a higher quality.*

- *Good quality vitamins have chelated minerals. This makes a huge difference in how well the minerals are absorbed by your body. For example, in supplements with calcium carbonate as its calcium source, less than 25% of the calcium is absorbed. In older adults, this absorption rate drops to about 10%. In contrast, if you take a supplement with calcium citrate (chelated), 30% - 50% of it is absorbed; almost twice as much! If you have any questions about specific supplements that you are taking, be sure to ask your chiropractor or nutritionist.*

- *Most good quality vitamin formulations require that you take more than one capsule or tablet per day. This is simply because good quality ingredients, such as chelated minerals, take up more space than their cheaper counterparts. Depending on your individual needs, you could be taking anywhere from two tablets per day for general nutritional support, to six tablets per day if you are an athlete or have special nutritional needs.*

- *Good quality vitamins will have adequate levels of biotin, whereas cheap, drugstore vitamins will not. Biotin is the most expensive vitamin to manufacture. Cheaper vitamins will have very little biotin in them compared to higher quality vitamins, and is one of the reasons why good vitamins cost a little more.*

Condition Specific Supplementation

In addition to taking a multivitamin, research has shown that certain natural supplements may be useful in the management of painful syndromes. Doctors of Chiropractic undergo extensive training in the area of nutrition and often prescribe nutritional support for their patients' specific needs.

Glucosamine Sulfate

Glucosamine sulfate has been used to successfully manage osteoarthritis for several years. Osteoarthritis is typically treated with analgesics, anti-inlammatories, and corticosteroids. Although often effective, these medications are not always tolerated well and long-term use can be dangerous. Glucosamine sulfate is known as a "chondroprotective" supplement, meaning it can be used to stop the evolution of osteoarthritis. This naturally occurring molecule, which is derived from shellfish, has been shown to have anti-inflammatory effects as well.

Glucosamine has been shown to result in longer term relief from pain when compared to non-steroidal anti-inflammatories (such as aspirin, ibuprofen, and naproxen). In November of 2005, a study at the University of Utah which looked at 1,583 patients with osteoarthritis, concluded that a glucosamine / chondroitin supplement performed as well, if not better, than Pfizer's Celebrex®. (*The Tan Sheet*, November 14, 2005).

Natural Muscle Relaxants

In some cases, the use of natural muscle relaxants will be useful for spasm, sprains, strains, muscle pulls, tension, soreness, or other muscle-related pain. Combinations of Valerian Root, Passion Flower, and Magnesium have been shown to be safe and may be effective for muscular pain. I often use a combination of these natural ingredients, known as Formula 303, for my patients.

A Final Thought on Nutrition

The foods you eat on a daily basis have a tremendous impact on your overall health. If you eat all-natural, health-giving foods, your body will be healthy. If you eat junk, your physical health will suffer. Remember that your body's only source for its building materials is the food that you eat.

In addition to eating a wide variety of natural, health-giving foods, it is also critical to take a good quality vitamin supplement and drink plenty of water. The vitamin supplement ensures that all of the metabolic processes in your body can be performed effectively and the water helps to keep the metabolic waste and toxins flushed out of your system.

When clinically appropriate for specific conditions, the use of safe and natural supplements may speed healing, minimize inflammation, and reduce pain. The entire realm of nutritional management for specific health conditions is beyond the scope of this book and takes up volumes. Turmeric, Boswellia, and other Ayurvedic herbs are showing promise as strong anti-inflammatories. The use of homeopathic treatment in chiropractic offices is not uncommon. Proteolytic enzymes may be useful in cases of acute injury.

As with any treatment recommendation, your doctor should be able to explain your nutritional options, as well as the latest research on the safety and effectiveness of anything he or she prescribes.

12

Ten Tips for a Healthier Lifestyle

"Health is defined as a state of complete physical, mental, and social well-being, and not merely the absence of disease or infirmity."

- The World Health Organization

Chiropractic is about more than back pain. As we have discussed, it is a holistic health care discipline that emphasizes wellness and prevention in addition to pain relief. By making the right lifestyle choices now, you have the potential to prevent health problems in the future.

The bad news it that nothing will guarantee that you will never suffer from back pain. Exercising, eating well, getting plenty of rest, and not smoking will certainly go a long way toward keeping your back healthy and pain-free, but back or neck pain, like the common cold, seem to hit just about everybody at one time or another.

Now for the good news: you can prevent most cases of back pain yourself with some simple stretches, exercises, and lifestyle changes. In fact, if you make these things a part of your daily routine, you can usually prevent back pain from occurring in the first place.

Maintain Good Posture

Poor posture creates excessive stress on your spine and can cause chronic muscle tension, leading to pain and stiffness. This happens because the weight of your upper body must be supported by your back muscles instead of the bones of your spine. The further your posture deviates from your center of gravity, the greater the stress on your back and the more pain that you will experience.

A simple exercise to improve your posture is called the Wall Posture Exercise. To do this exercise, simply find a flat wall. Rest your back against the wall and scoot your heels, shoulders, and head back until they touch the wall. Holding this posture, step away from the wall and try to hold this posture as long as you can while you go about your day.

Reduce Your Stress

Although it is generally accepted that emotional stress or psychological factors can make any back pain problem worse, the concept of "stress-related" back pain takes this idea one step further. The diagnosis of stress-related back pain assumes that psychological and emotional factors are of primary influence.

The stress-related back pain diagnosis is a "psychosomatic" or "psycho-physiological" one. A psycho-physiological illness is any illness in which physical symptoms are thought to be the direct result of psychological or emotional factors. This diagnosis means that psychological factors either initiated or are maintaining the back pain, or both.

It should be emphasized that even though psychological factors may be causing the physical symptoms, the symptoms are not imaginary. They are very real physical problems (such as back pain), which are being impacted upon by emotional factors.

Such practices as daily meditation, prayer, or yoga may help you relax and minimize the effects of a stressful life.

Maintain a Healthy Body Weight

Most people know that excessive body weight contributes to the development of a number of conditions such as coronary heart disease, diabetes, high blood pressure, and colon cancer. However, it may also be a major contributing factor for the development of low back pain. The spine is designed to carry a certain amount of body weight. When it is exposed to the excess pressure of being overweight, the spine becomes stressed and, over time, can suffer structural damage. Being overweight significantly contributes to symptoms associated with osteoporosis, osteoarthritis (OA), rheumatoid arthritis (RA), degenerative disc disease (DDD), spinal stenosis, and spondylolisthesis.

In addition to back pain, those who are overweight may suffer from fatigue as well as difficulty breathing and shortness of breath during short periods of exercise. If the fatigue and shortness of breath cause one to avoid activity and exercise, then this can indirectly lead to back pain.

If you are currently overweight and suffer from low back pain, talk to your doctor about effective ways to lose weight. Not only will your back pain decrease, but you will lower your risk of most major degenerative diseases at the same time.

Sleep on a Good Mattress

Good health and sleep are closely linked. Just as we improve our eating habits for better health, we should also improve our sleep habits. Sleep should be a priority and not just a negotiable need determined by our busy schedules. Good sleep not only reduces costly back problems but also helps to prepare us for a more productive, alert, and safe day ahead.

Here are some tips to help you select the proper mattress for you:

- Personal preference should ultimately determine what mattress to purchase. Any mattress that helps someone sleep without pain and stiffness is the best mattress for that individual. There is no single mattress that works for all people with low back pain.

- Find a mattress with sufficient back support to reduce low back pain. A good mattress should provide support while allowing for the natural curves and alignment of the spine. Medium-firm mattresses usually provide more back pain relief than firm mattresses.

- Know when it's time to get a new mattress. If an old mattress sags visibly in the middle, it is probably time to purchase a new one. Putting boards under a sagging mattress is only a short-term fix and may cause more back problems and low back pain in the long run.

• Be wary of mattress advertising gimmicks. Claims that a mattress is "orthopedic" or "medically-approved" should be viewed skeptically. There has not been extensive medical research or controlled clinical trials on the topic of mattresses and low back pain. You must determine whether or not extra features on a mattress make it more comfortable or supportive for your back.

Wear Orthotics

Orthotics are custom fitted inserts that you place into your shoes to keep your feet functioning correctly. Your feet are the foundation of your body. They support you when you stand, walk, or run. They also help protect your spine, bones, and soft tissues from damaging stress as you move around. Your feet perform better when all their muscles, arches, and bones are in their ideal stable positions.

The foot is constructed with three arches which, when properly maintained, give exceptional supportive strength. These three arches form a supporting vault that distributes the weight of the entire body. If there is compromise of one arch in the foot, the other arches must compensate and are subject to additional stresses, which usually leads to further compromise.

By stabilizing and balancing your feet, orthotics enhance your body's performance and efficiency, reduce pain, and contribute to your total body wellness. Since the average person spends almost two-thirds of their day in shoes, it's important to make sure that they provide optimal support. The particular brand of orthotics that I recommend are called Foot Levelers. Foot Levelers orthotics support all three arches in your feet, thereby creating a stable foundation upon which to build proper body posture.

Drink More Water

Water is the single-most abundant nutrient in the body, accounting for around 60% - 65% of your total weight. It is also the least forgiving of all the nutrients you consume. You can survive for weeks without food but for only a couple of days without water. Water is responsible for the transport of nutrients, oxygen, and waste products, as well as for regulating your body temperature and serving as the medium in which all of your body's chemical reactions take place. Most people do not drink enough pure clean water.

Drinking an adequate amount of clean water every day is one of the most overlooked but simplest ways of keeping your body healthy. Water is used to help the body cleanse itself of toxins and metabolic waste. Although drinking water has become more popular over the past several years, many people still do not consume enough water. Instead, they drink coffee, tea, juices, and soft drinks and figure that they get enough fluids. It is true that when you drink these things you are consuming water. However, along with the water, you are also consuming other substances that the body will need to ultimately eliminate, so the potential beneficial effect of the water is somewhat negated. To make matters worse, drinks that contain caffeine such as coffee, tea, and soft drinks actually cause more water loss than the amount of water they contain, resulting in a net loss of water.

Ideally, the average person should consume around ten cups of water per day, or just over a half gallon. Some of this water is found in the food and beverages you consume, so you don't have to drink an entire half-gallon of water every day. What I tell my patients to do is to buy a 1.5 liter bottle of water from the local grocery store and to drink that amount of water every day. If you exercise heavily, you may have to drink two of those 1.5 liter bottles of water each day. By drinking enough water, you will be helping your body to remain healthy. It is by far the cheapest health insurance you can buy.

Eat More Fruits and Vegetables

People know that they should eat more fruit and vegetables in their diet, but most people don't. Lately it seems that the four major food groups of the American diet have gone from dairy, fruits and vegetables, grains and meat to sugar, fat, salt, and caffeine. Because of the easy availability of fast foods and snack foods, we have lost our taste for fruits and vegetables, especially vegetables. It is not uncommon for many people to go for weeks without consuming a single serving of fresh vegetables. This is not good.

The human body evolved with a diet high in fruits and vegetables and is dependent on many of the compounds unique to plant foods in order to operate correctly. If you don't consume enough of these plant compounds, your energy level will suffer along with your overall health. Most people are shocked at how much better they feel when they cut down on fast foods and snack foods and increase their fruit and vegetable intake.

If you find it difficult to work in several servings of fruits and vegetables into your routine every day, you may find it helpful to supplement your diet with what is called a "greens" supplement, which is a highly concentrated powder of fruits, vegetables, and antioxidants.

Increasing your consumption of fruits and vegetables is an important way to improve your overall health. The key is to make it part of your lifestyle - to make it a new habit.

Keep Your Heart Healthy

Heart disease is currently the number-one killer of adults in the United States. This is unfortunate because most heart disease is caused by poor lifestyle choices. The four big lifestyle changes you can make to ensure to maximize the health of your heart are exercise, maintaining a healthy body weight, taking a high quality vitamin supplement, and stopping smoking.

Just as exercise is important to the health of your neuromusculoskeletal system, it is also critical to the health of your heart. When you regularly exercise, your body becomes much more efficient at using oxygen and burning calories and your blood pressure is normalized. This decreases the stress on your heart.

Another easy way to reduce the stress on your heart is to decrease the amount of body fat you carry around. It takes approximately one mile of additional blood vessels to supply one pound of additional fat. If you are twenty, thirty, or fifty pounds overweight, it is easy to see how that extra body fat can place an undue burden on your heart.

Vitamins E, C, and folic acid are the three most important nutritional supplements for your heart. Vitamin E is a powerful fat-soluble antioxidant which helps to prevent the cholesterol in your blood from becoming oxidized. High cholesterol levels in the blood, per se, are not that big of a deal. Cholesterol only becomes dangerous when it interacts with an oxidizing radical. Vitamin E helps to prevent this.

Vitamin C is important to help strengthen the walls of the arteries and prevent the development of cholesterol plaques inside the coronary arteries. Did you know that the arteries that are the most likely to develop cholesterol deposits are the ones that are close to the heart? The reason is that when the heart contracts, it pushes blood out with a great degree of force. If the walls of the arteries which are closest to the heart are not as strong as they should be, they will tend to momentarily stretch out like a balloon and cause small tears to the inside arterial wall as the rush of blood from the heart passes by. These small tears serve as a place where platelets and cholesterol form deposits. High levels of vitamin C reduce the number of tears in the arteries by strengthening the collagen tissues around the arteries, keeping them from expanding too much as blood pulses through.

The third vitamin which is important is one of the B-vitamins called folic acid. Folic acid, also called folacin, is important for reducing the level of homocysteine in the blood. Homocysteine is a metabolic by-product which can contribute significantly to the development of heart disease.

So, when you take your multivitamin while you are on your way to do your exercises, make sure that it contains at least 400 IU of vitamin E, at least 500 mg of vitamin C (1000 is even better), and 40 mcg of folic acid.

Lift Correctly

There is no single lifting technique that will work in every situation. Lifting a small heavy box off of the floor requires a very different technique than lifting a canoe up onto the roof of your van. For this reason, it's better to learn the five basic rules for safe lifting: keep the load in front of you, minimize bending at the waist, keep the load close to your body, take a wide stance, and get help with large items. Let's take a look at each one of these rules and why they are important for reducing your risk of low back injury.

• Keep the load in front of you. The bones and muscles of the body have their maximum strength in the center of the body and are weaker and more prone to injury on the sides. This is why you should never twist when you are lifting.

• Minimize bending at the waist. The low back is a very mobile area of the body. Unfortunately, this degree of mobility also makes it more unstable and susceptible to injury than most other parts of the body. Frequent bending at the waist is a very common cause of low back injury because bending at the waist places all of the stress from the weight of your upper body as well as the weight of the item you are lifting directly onto the unstable low back. To reduce the risk of low back injury, you will want to minimize the amount of bending you have to do when lifting. This can be accomplished by bending more at the knees when you have to lift something off the floor and,whenever possible, to position the load at waist-level before lifting it.

• Keep the load close to your body. The closer that you can keep the load to your center of gravity, the less strain it will be on your body. Keeping the load close decreases the stress on your low back and reduces your chance of injury.

• Take a wide stance. By taking a wide stance when you have to lift something, it is easier to keep the load closer to your center of gravity, thereby minimizing the stress on your back. It minimizes the amount of bending at the waist by allowing you to keep your hips under your body and it allows you to use the strong muscles of the legs and buttocks to help you lift, rather than the weaker muscles of the low back.

• Get help when lifting large items. Every year, many people are injured when they attempt to lift too much. The object that they try to lift may not even be too heavy, it may just be too large. A large light-weight box can put as much stress on the back as a small heavy box. Ask someone to help you with heavy or awkward items.

Stop Smoking

Bone is a living tissue dependent on the functions and support provided by the other body systems. When these systems are not able to perform normally, bone is unable to rebuild itself. The formation of bone is particularly influenced by physical exercise and hormonal activity, both of which are adversely affected by cigarette smoking.

Smoking reduces the amount of oxygen in the blood and increases the level of harmful substances such as carbon monoxide. In addition, nicotine causes a constriction of the small blood vessels that feed your spinal discs, shutting down their nutrient supply. Over time, the loss of normal blood supply leads to your discs becoming dehydrated, and they begin to degenerate. Smoking is also known to cause an increase in estrogen loss in women who are perimenopausal or postmenopausal, which can result in a loss of bone density and increase your risk of developing osteoporosis.

There is no question that it is difficult to quit smoking. Many people who have quit say that it was the hardest thing they have ever done. However, it is not impossible; people do it all the time. If you currently smoke and want to quit, there are a number of effective medical programs that can help you. Some people have also found complimentary therapies, such as hypnosis, to be helpful in quitting smoking.

A New Paradigm in Health Care

Unlocking the Spinal Code: Doctor and Patient as a Healthcare Team

Doctors have a responsibility to educate their patients, make recommendations based on solid medical evidence, and administer safe and effective therapies. However, true progress in the management of spinal pain does not only involve treatments that are done to you (known as passive treatment) by a doctor or therapist, but also activities performed by you (known as active care).

Quitting smoking, following your doctor's advice, losing weight, exercising, keeping scheduled appointments, eating a healthy diet, praying, meditating, and asking questions and learning about your problem and treatments is encouraged and necessary for true progress.

I always emphasize the team approach between doctor and patient in managing back pain. My patients are confident that I will do all that I can to provide them with quality care. In return, however, I expect positive lifestyle changes that will enhance healing and overall wellness. True progress in managing back pain occurs when there is a synergistic formula of active and passive care.

Much like a finely tuned car, your body requires maintenance in the form of exercise, proper nutrition and diet, regular chiropractic adjustments, and positive lifestyle changes. By maintaining this "vehicle" now, you will minimize the need for more drastic interventions later.

When treatment for spinal pain is necessary, you can be confident that Doctors of Chiropractic are highly trained in diagnosis and management. Integrated Spine Care Centers, which include spine specialists from different disciplines, also offer a beacon of hope for effective chronic pain management by utilizing various treatments and interventions. The "team" of doctor and patient is broadened when various practitioners work together for the benefit of the patient.

By returning to this book as a reference in the future, you will possess an understanding of and an appreciation for the human body, and the spine in particular. You are now armed with a body of knowledge that will guide you in the pursuit of a healthy, pain-free lifestyle.

"The great end of life is not knowledge, but action."

- Thomas Huxley

About Dr. Douglas Jay Taber

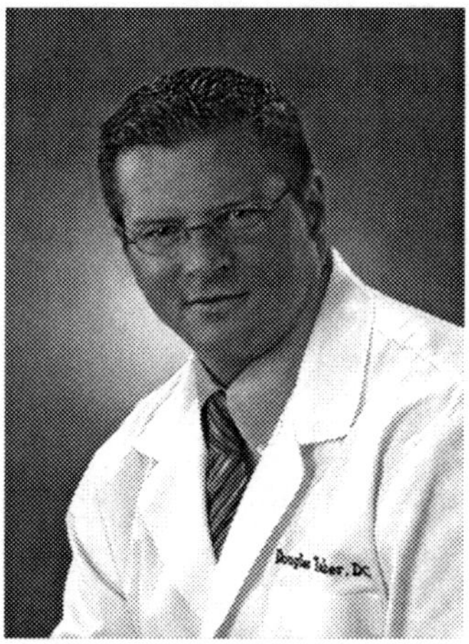

Dr. Douglas Taber is a nationally recognized expert in the diagnosis and treatment of spine-related disorders. He is a 1998 graduate of New York Chiropractic College and holds a Bachelor of Science degree from the State University of New York at Fredonia. He is a former Certified Personal Trainer with the National Strength & Conditioning Association.

Dr. Taber is Board Certified in Pain Management by the American Academy of Experts in Traumatic Stress and is a Diplomate of the American Academy of Pain Management, which is a multidisciplinary international academy of 7000 pain practitioners worldwide. He has also achieved status as a Diplomate of the American Academy of Experts in Traumatic Stress. He is a Fellow of the American Academy of Chiropractic Physicians.

Dr. Taber is a Diplomate of the College of Physicians and a Fellow of the American Association of Integrative Medicine. He is the first Doctor of Chiropractic to achieve Diplomate status with the American Association of Spine Physicians. Dr. Taber is Certified in Manipulation Under Anesthesia and is a member of the National Academy of MUA Physicians.

Dr. Taber is a Fellow of the American Back Society and a Fellow of the American Board of Disability Analysts. He is a Certified Ergonomics Technician, a Certified Independent Chiropractic Examiner with the National Board of Independent Medical Examiners, and a member of the American College of Forensic Examiners.

In 1998, Dr. Taber was the recipient of the BJ Palmer Award for his literary contributions to the chiropractic profession. In 2004, he was selected as "One of America's Top Chiropractors" by the Consumer Research Council of America. He has recently been nominated as "International Health Professional of 2006" for his contributions to spine care.

Dr. Taber maintains a private practice in the Southern Tier of New York and is Director of Chiropractic Services at the Southern Tier Pain Management Center and Conservative Care Director at the Binghamton Spine Care Center. He lectures extensively to health care providers and the general public on the evidence-based non-surgical treatment of spinal disorders and overall health and wellness.

For more information on Dr. Taber, chiropractic care, and spinal health, visit our website at

www.chiropracticassociates.info

- Order Form -

The Back Pain Solution
Unlocking the Spinal Code

Please mail or fax this form to

Dr. Douglas Jay Taber
200 Front Street • Vestal, NY 13850
fax: (607) 754-1477

Name: ______________________________

Address: ______________________________

____

City: ________________ State: ______ Zip: __________

Phone: ________________ Fax: ________________

Quantity: __________

Subtotal ($14.95 per book): __________

Shipping ($2.00 per book): __________

Total: __________

Payment method:

☐ Check enclosed ☐ VISA ☐ MasterCard ☐ Discover

Name as it appears on card: ______________________________

Card #: ________________ Exp: ______ Verification #: ______

I hereby authorize that my credit card be charged for the total due for this order.

Signature: ______________________________ Date: __________

Printed in the United States
49584LVS00001BA/124-186